I have spent many years following my [...] to listen to the cultural talk that led n[...] confused mind. Then I heard a voice with strong words and a movement practice to back it up. *Change Your Body, Change the World* will open a path to making sense of the predicament of our time. It's an invitation that inspires all of us to learn the craft and cultivate our organic body with the organics of the land. If you desire a change in yourself and in the way we relate to the world, then pick up this book—walk, run, dance, lift, swing and play each essay as part of your training and remember.

    Mick Dodge
    The Barefoot Sensei

Frank's prose is deeply authentic. He has a deep insight into the human predicament—where we go wrong and how we can rectify it. Frank's wisdom comes from a lifetime of contemplating and experiencing real life and he understands 'the human' in his bones. This is no removed academic piece, it is a book of visceral honest love for our place in nature and it throws us a challenge that we can't ignore.

    Tara Wood
    Founder of Wildfitness

Frank Forencich is blessed with that rare long-range vision required to see how seemingly disparate pieces actually fit together. In *Change Your Body, Change The World*, Frank continues the work he began with *Play As If Your Life Depends On It* and *Exuberant Animal*, brilliantly illuminating and linking the essential points of our physical reality with logic, common sense and (of course) playful humor. Consume this book like a great multi-course feast.

    Steve Myrland
    Myrland Sports Training
    Beacon Athletics

This book is transformative, especially with regard to the connections between society, mental health, environmental health, and movement. As someone who works with children and counsels families on a daily basis, Frank's thoughts on the influence of culture and environment on health ring truer than ever.

>Dr. Kwame M. Brown
>Child development specialist and youth fitness consultant

Frank Forencich has emerged as one of the most thoughtful and insightful action-based philosophers on human movement. In this collection of essays, the reader is treated to a meditation on the functional aspect of play in human development, and provoked with a reflection on the "tyranny of technology" that causes the "body/world problem." This is not a how-to book: Forencich's agenda is more bold and ambitious than the empty promise of a lifestyle makeover. Rather, he inspires us to critically wrestle with our place in the world.

>J.R. Atwood
>Social scientist and founder of Playthink

At a time when our society looks to genetic engineering and pharmacological interventions to improve our health, Frank Forencich reminds us that the most essential keys to healthy minds and bodies are right outside our windows. Through millions of years of evolution, the human body and brain have been fine-tuned to respond optimally to the natural environment—to dirt, wind, rain, physical challenges, and complex face-to-face social interactions. *Change Your Body, Change the World* forces us to consider the natural costs of our technological, sedentary lifestyles. After reading this book, you'll view our society's many "advances" in a new light and will opt for "real" encounters with nature.

>Kelly G. Lambert, Ph.D.
>Macon and Joan Brock Professor of
>Psychology, Randolph-Macon College
>President, International Behavioral Neuroscience Society

CHANGE YOUR BODY, CHANGE THE WORLD

REFLECTIONS ON HEALTH AND THE HUMAN PREDICAMENT

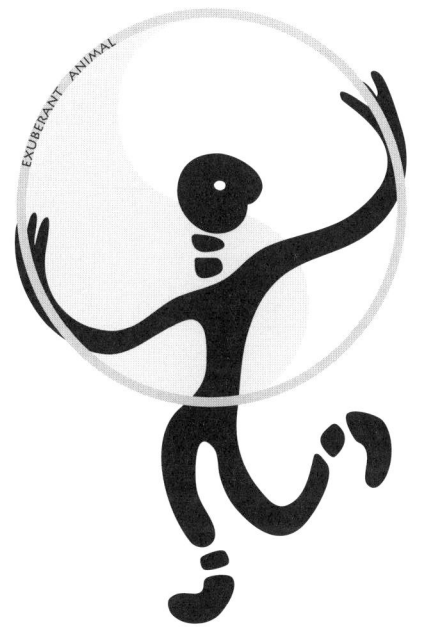

FRANK FORENCICH

AN EXUBERANT ANIMAL® PUBLICATION

© 2010 Exuberant Animal®. All rights reserved. No part of this book may be reproduced or transmitted in any form or by any means—except by a reviewer who may quote brief passages in a review—without permission in writing from the publisher. For information, contact Exuberant Animal at 9112 32nd Ave. NE, Seattle, WA 98115.

ISBN 0-9723358-5-4

Library of Congress Control Number: 2010929021

Printed in the United States of America

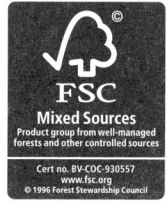

PRINTED ON FSC-CERTIFIED PAPER

Forest Stewardship Council (FSC) is a non-profit organization devoted to encouraging the responsible management of the world's forests. FSC sets high standards that ensure forestry is practiced in an environmentally responsible, socially beneficial, and economically viable way.

Trusted environmental organizations including Greenpeace, National Wildlife Federation, The Nature Conservancy, Sierra Club, and World Wildlife Fund all support and encourage FSC certification. Consumers wishing to support healthy forests and communities should look and ask for the FSC label when purchasing wood or paper products. For more information about FSC, please visit www.fsc.org.

WARNING

Before beginning a program of sedentary living and isolation from the natural world, see your physician, your therapist and your insurance agent. While you're at it, check with your family and friends. You are about to embark on a perilous lifestyle that is dangerous not only to yourself, but also to those around you.

A truly good book teaches me better than to read it. I must soon lay it down, and commence living on its hint. What I began by reading, I must finish by acting.

                        Henry David Thoreau

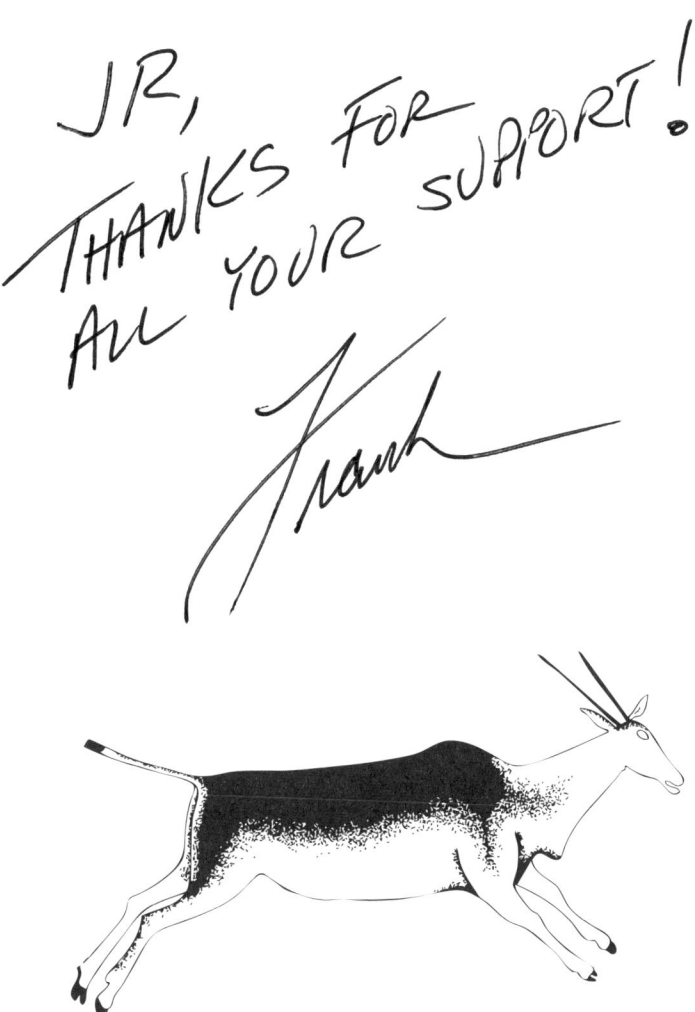

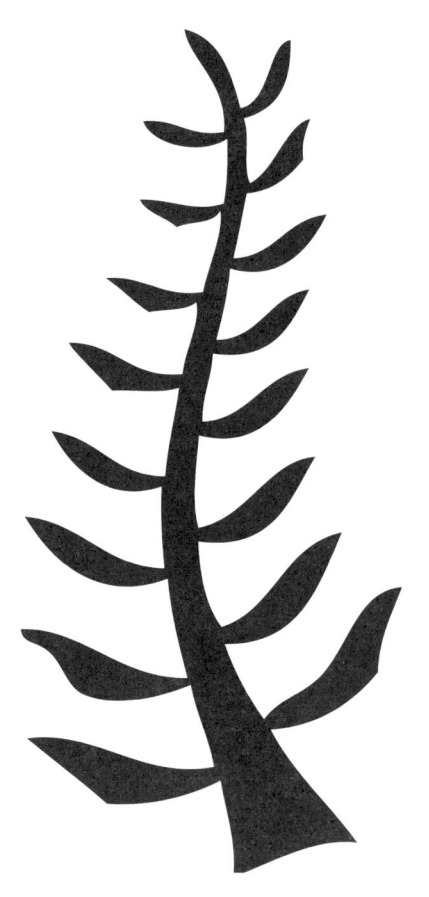

CONTENTS

THE BODY IS VAST 1

PANORAMA 7

BODY TALK
    Primate's predicament 19
    The first thing that happens 29
    No body is an island 35
    Primal confusion 43
    See the light 49
    The case against exercise 53
    Pumped to perfection 59
    The art of the arc 67
    Romancing the body 75

TAKE A CULTURE
    Cogito ergo dumb 83
    Pathology on parade 89
    I know it when i see it 95
    Dojo rules 103
    Robots are from mars, humans are from earth 109
    We interrupt this broadcast 115

LIFEWAYS

Let's see... 121
Life on the mississippi 129
Learning from the inside out 133
Playstate 137
Welcome to the neo-paleo 145
Digital mastery 153
Comic relief 159

CHANGE YOUR BODY, CHANGE THE WORLD

The first rule of navigation 169
The future is plastic 177
Playing in the shadow of the beast 181
Rapport reform 187
Embodied solutions 195
Rut craft 203
Earth lust 211
Bag of tricks 219

ACTION STEPS   225

RECOMMENDED READING   227

THE PRIMAL SCHOLAR   231

WORKSHOPS   233

THE BODY IS VAST

> We are ignorant about how we work, about where we fit in, and most of all about the enormous, imponderable system of life in which we are embedded as working parts. We do not really understand nature, at all.
>
> Lewis Thomas
> *Lives of a Cell*

Opinions about the body are like bodies—everybody's got one. We're all intimately familiar with the experience of living in a body and almost everyone believes that they know what they're talking about. We live in our bodies all day, every day and we're quick to suppose that we understand what they are and how they work.

It's an easy trap to fall into of course, but our presumption of understanding erodes at an astonishing rate when we begin to study the body in depth. After a few years of looking at the myriad relationships in and around the body, the familiar starts to look incredible, beautiful, and on some days, completely miraculous. The deeper we look, the more detail we see, the more dynamism we discover and the more astounding the totality becomes. Finally, just as we feel that we're about to grasp the thing itself, we realize that we know almost nothing about it. Ultimately, there's only one appropriate reaction to a deep study of the human body and that is *awe*.

Even the short story is incredible: Each of us is home to some 10 trillion somatic cells, each one a marvel of sophistication in its own right. Within each nucleus lie some 25,000 genes, layered with powerful epigenetic mechanisms that turn genes on and off in response to environmental conditions. At a macro level, we are home to dozens of organs, hundreds of bones and muscles, the whole system orchestrated by a nervous system of dizzying intricacy—dozens of neurotransmitters and uncountable billions of synapses, each in a dynamic dance of growth and decay.

If this was the full extent of our physical complexity, we might be able to get our minds around the body, so to speak. But this inventory of component parts, mind-blowing as it is, is only the simple stuff. The real complications come into play when we begin to understand that all this complexity is massively influenced by personal history, psychology and placebo effects. Belief can have a profound impact on our physical experience and in turn, the function and structure of our bodies.

Even if we could somehow comprehend the effects of individual beliefs on individual bodies, we're still left with the confounding influences of society and culture. As we're now beginning to realize, socio-cultural effects on health can be powerful and highly contagious. In a very real way, our bodies don't even belong entirely to us; to some degree, we actually create one another as we live our lives together. And if our bodies are all linked and interdependent, how will we ever sort out the chain of causality?

Will Durant once observed that "Education is the progressive discovery of your own ignorance." Nowhere is this truer than in matters of the body. It is even more the case when we attempt to study the body in a larger context of natural history, environment and culture. And so it is that I've come to this investigation of the body and the earth, filled with a sense of awe and a nagging, persistent awareness of my ignorance. Fortunately, I belong to a tribe of truly exceptional friends and colleagues who have helped me to hold my own against the forces of confusion and complexity:

Dawni Rae and Alia Joy Bugaboo Shaw, the light of your love has blessed me beyond measure. Sam Forencich, rock of dependable counsel and good humor. Stuart Brown, inspiring mentor and guide. Kwame Brown, co-conspirator in mischief and social activism. Sebastien Alary, extraordinary mountain partner. Susan Fahringer, grounded friend for life. Jeri Helen, expert wordsmith and guardian of language. Jamie Wheal and the EA Alchemists: Josh Leeger, Charlie Reid and Colin Pistell. Tara Wood, Edward Drax and the tribe at Wildfitness.

Other exuberants have stepped up as well: Dave Wilson, Jackie Endsley, Scott McCredie, Martha Peterson, Skye Nacel, Steve Myrland, Mary Collins, Steve Laskevitch, Gary Avischious, Mariah Burton Nelson, J.R. Atwood, Kelly Lambert, Wolf Brolley, Danny McMillian, Erwan Le Corre and Barefoot Ted.

And finally, a special appreciation to my friend and teacher, the Barefoot Sensei. You are a wise guide and powerful visionary; your walk and your talk are strong. My gratitude is immense.

MISMATCH

> It may well be that more and more of what people bring before doctors and therapists for treatment—agonies of body and spirit—are symptoms of the biospheric emergency registering at the most intimate levels of life. The Earth hurts, and we hurt with it.
>
> Theodore Roszak
> *The Voice of the Earth*

The year was 1962, the setting a small alpine valley near Lake Tahoe in the Sierra Nevada Mountains of California. I was but a young creature, a curious mammal of no particular distinction. It was a glorious summer day and my first real exposure to an alpine habitat. Our family was camped beside the Carson River and for the first time, I was cut loose to explore the banks of a nearly pristine mountain stream.

My mother kept a vigilant watch as I scrambled up, down and along the stream bank. I soon discovered the boulders—gorgeous granite blocks that were both smooth and rough, clean and inviting. As I climbed and scrambled, I had the most powerful realization of my young life, a personal Zen moment that has stayed with me for almost 50 years.

At first contact with the granite, I was overcome with pleasure as my hands, feet and knees touched the gorgeous orbs. I was instantly delighted with a profound sense of exuberance—astonished that something could feel so good and so right for my body. My muscles rejoiced; these shapes were perfect for pushing, pulling, climbing and jumping. It was like the playground at my elementary school, only a thousand times better. It struck me as a wonderful coincidence: these boulders, this river—this world—was made just for me, for my body. Or, I was made for it. But no matter; every detail of the outer world seemed a ideal match with every detail of my anatomy and physiology. My joy was boundless; I belonged to this place. My body, mind and spirit were happy.

Not surprisingly, the boulders continued to draw me back, even after my family returned home to what would later be called Silicon Valley. As my body matured, I returned to the Sierras at every opportunity and touched the alpine habitat in every way possible: hiking, scrambling and climbing the walls in Yosemite. I loved the granitic world and it loved me back. My body became strong and my spirit soared.

But sadly, the joy of my first alpine contact was later eclipsed by an equal and opposite experience, a toxic event that has repeated itself thousands of times over my adult life. This time I was stuck in traffic somewhere south of Oakland, boxed in by a pod of monstrous 18-wheelers, incarcerated in a cage of sheet metal, glass and plastic. The summertime heat was intense and the exhaust savaged my lungs and eyes. All I could see were cars, trucks, concrete retaining walls and outdoor advertising—no plants, no animals, no color, no texture. Not only was my world lifeless, noisy and hostile, I was utterly powerless to change it or escape. Stress hormones flooded my bloodstream and my spirit raged.

I sought refuge in the radio, but all I could hear were annoying advertisements and yet more noise. As I fought back against my predicament, a voice rose up through the stress of my frantic consciousness: "My body is not made for this! This place is not made for my body." My tissue screamed, "This is profoundly, fundamentally wrong. It is wrong by a million years. It is a mismatch for every cell of my being; I hate it and I am right to hate it."

Unfortunately, there have been many such instances of environmental mismatch in my adult life, days in which the moments of distress and alienation far outnumber the Zen moments of perfect fit. Increasingly, as modernity grows ever more tyrannical, my sense of psychophysical alienation grows as well.

This experience is much more than my own neurotic drama, however. My sense of mismatch is now shared by an increasing number of people around the world. We may not put it precisely in these terms, but our bodies know the truth: our modern world is an increasingly unfriendly and alien place. Something is drastically, spectacularly wrong with the world that we have created.

For some, this connection between personal and environmental health is an abstraction; they see no association between a sick biosphere and a sick body. They feel terrible, but can't say why. They see no relationship between the pain in their bodies and the accelerating destruction of habitat around the world. Others are more sensitive to large-scale planetary influences. Dave Foreman, founder of Earth First!, describes his experience this way:

> I am an animal! A living being of flesh and blood, storm and fury. The oceans of the Earth course through my veins, the winds of the sky fill my lungs, the very bedrock of the planet makes my bones. I am alive! When a chain saw slices into the heartwood of a two-thousand year old Coast Redwood, it's slicing into my guts. When a bulldozer rips through the Amazon rain forest, it's ripping into my side. When a Japanese whaler fires an exploding harpoon into a great whale, my heart is blown to smithereens. I am the land, the land is me.

This is not just the poetic raving of a frustrated activist. Say what you will about Dave Foreman and his utopian band of Earth First! eco-criminals, I have no question that Mr. Foreman literally feels these things in his body. I also have no question that these events are likely to have adverse effects on his health and our health as well.

Over the last several decades, many people have had experiences similar to Dave Foreman's and my own. Many of us have felt the extreme physical distress of the body–environment mismatch. Locked in climate-controlled buildings, working around the clock, stuck in cars, eating food-like substances of unknowable origins, living in ambiguous networks of constantly shifting alliances, our bodies begin to squirm, our teeth begin to grind and our spirits suffer. Disease creeps into our tissue.

We write off our anxiety in various ways. Perhaps it is our fault for being unhappy in this modern world. Perhaps we are maladjusted; maybe we need psychotherapy or medication. Perhaps a doctor can help us feel better. Maybe some alternative methods will get us back on track. Maybe we just need to train harder and push through the adversity.

But increasingly, many of us are beginning to realize that, in one sense, it's not our fault at all. We feel an incredible sense of physical and psychological angst, not because there's anything wrong with us, but because there is something profoundly wrong with the world we have created for ourselves. We are OK; it's our human-engineered environment that's killing us.

If you've been suffering this deep primal angst, this sense of environmental–existential pathology, you are not alone. In fact, your suspicions are now being validated by scientists across the spectrum. Paleontologists, evolutionary biologists, physicians, psychologists, zoologists and animal behavior specialists are all beginning to see our predicament with greater clarity. All animals, including humans, do best in their native environment. Change that environment drastically—as we have done—and you're bound to see distress. It doesn't matter whether you're fish or fowl, buffalo or biped: life in a mismatched habitat is bound to be difficult for flesh and for spirit.

The good news is that the body is set to make a comeback, and not a moment too soon. For centuries the human body has been locked up in a Cartesian prison, stifled by a Puritan-Victorian value system, punished by workaholism, pushed off the land and isolated from the natural world. We've disempowered ourselves by putting our bodies into the hands of a professional expert class. We've medicalized every dimension of physical living: birth, exercise, food and death. We've professionalized youth sports and taken away recess for both children and adults. The body has been incarcerated by its own hand and is now beginning to suffer the consequences in epidemic levels of psychophysical disease and unhappiness: obesity, heart disease, diabetes, depression and physical apathy.

But there's a change in the air and on the ground. The body's comeback is being driven by discoveries in neuroscience and social psychology that prove beyond question that the body is deeply and intimately involved at every level of human experience. These discoveries tell us something that is at once ridiculously obvious and profoundly counter-cultural: the body is essential to our lives. Its health is crucially important to the vitality and function of the brain, to social cohesion, creativity, decision-making and in turn, to prosperity and a sustainable human future. It has now become clear that our conventional "brain on a stick" approach to education, management and living is outmoded, ineffective and extremely dangerous.

It's time for the body to get back into the act.

PANORAMA

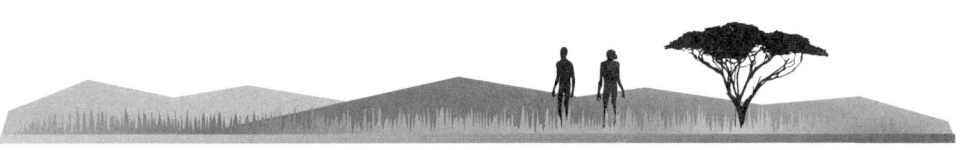

Change Your Body, Change the World

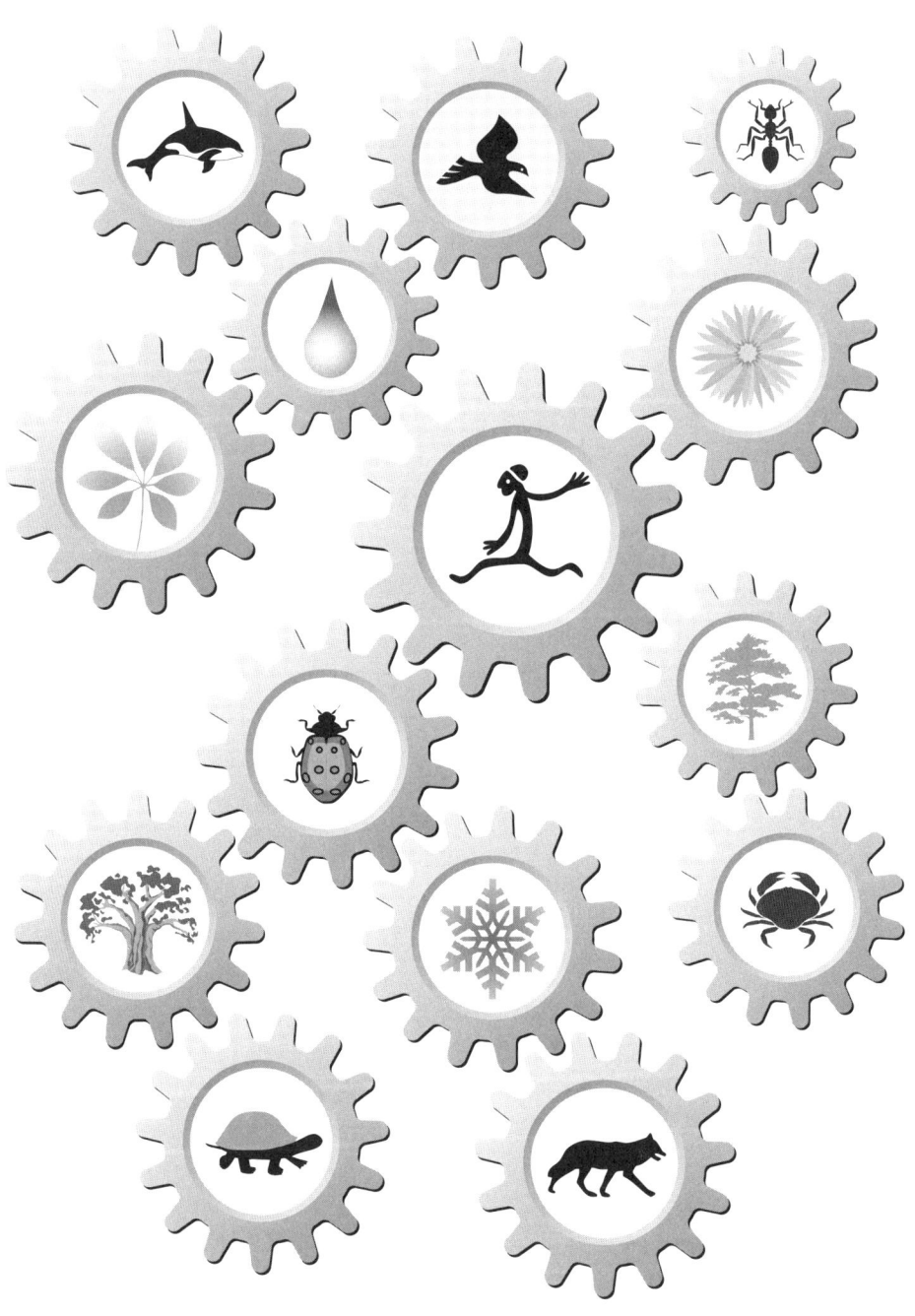

Change Your Body, Change the World

THE VERY FIRST THING

> I am I plus my surroundings, and if I do not preserve the latter, I do not preserve myself.
>
> Jose Ortega y Gasset

So, you want to change your body? Of course you do. Almost everyone in today's world has some sort of complaint about the state of their body: too fat, too slow, too weak, too funny-looking, too painful. Many of us feel uncomfortable, alienated, isolated and physically unhappy. The human body has become a focal point of discontent and suffering, both real and manufactured.

It's no surprise, of course. We're bombarded with reminders of our physical inadequacies throughout the day, each one drawing attention to our flaws and encouraging us to shape up. The messages are incessant: We need to be skinnier, younger and more muscular. We need to be skinnier, stronger and faster. We need to be more athletic, more stylish, sexier and above all, skinnier.

So, we gather up our resolve, drag ourselves off the couch and look around for a path. But where do we begin? What do we need to get started on the road to health?

It's a common question and lots of experts are standing by to provide the ultimate answer. Depending on what we read, we might discover that we need:

- a doctor's clearance
- a good pair of running shoes
- a gym membership
- a yoga mat and a fashionable set of lycra
- a water bottle and a box of supplements
- an electronic gadget with a software solution

Unfortunately, all of these answers are wrong. Not only are they wrong, they also distract us from our most fundamental need in the quest for health and physical happiness. That is, if we want to get started on a program for improving our health, the first thing that we need is *a functional habitat*.

Habitat is every animal's life support system. It provides our air, food and water, as well as a sense of identity and meaning. We are completely, utterly dependent upon it. Without a healthy, functioning habitat, there can be no fitness, no athletic excellence, no wellness and no sex appeal. There can be no exuberance, no happiness and ultimately, no life.

In the end, the fundamental principle is as simple as it is stark: *no habitat, no health*. If your life support system doesn't work, your body isn't going to work either, no matter how sophisticated your training program might happen to be. If the biosphere is sick, we are going to be sick as well. If we can't solve our problems of habitat, all the health advice in the world is worthless.

Clearly, our predicament calls for an integrated approach, one that puts the body into context and supports our efforts from both ends of the spectrum. What we need is an orientation that honors both the personal and the global, the physical and the ecological. The age of isolation and separation is over.

WELCOME TO "BIG HEALTH"

This book is a tale of two predicaments. On one hand, our bodies are suffering with an incredible burden of disease, dysfunction and unhappiness. Obesity, diabetes, heart disease, cancer and depression are ravaging the human body. These afflictions, described by the World Health Organization as non-communicable diseases (NCDs), now account for an immense disease burden worldwide. And even among people who are not strictly "diseased," there is a widespread sense of psychophysical suffering and anxiety.

At the same time, we are face-to-face with an unprecedented global ecological breakdown. Habitat is disintegrating all around us. Biodiversity is shrinking before our eyes and natural systems are eroding at a terrifying pace.

Some readers might wonder what these two domains have to do with one another. What does personal health have to do with the state of the world? Why should my fitness, obesity, diabetes, lethargy or depression have anything to do with global warming, oil spills, destruction of rainforests and oceans or the loss of biodiversity? Why should a health and fitness book have anything to say about ecosystems, biodiversity or habitat? Isn't health and fitness something that happens in a gym or a studio?

Conventional approaches address these two domains independently, as if personal health and environmental health were two entirely different specializations; In conventional practice, doctors work on bodies and biologists work on habitat. But in fact, these two realms are massively interconnected and interdependent. There is a powerful relationship between the way we experience our bodies and the way we relate to the wider world. The process works in both directions, for better and for worse.

This understanding and appreciation for human–habitat interdependence leads us towards an orientation I call "Big Health." Instead of seeing humans as a stand-alone, isolated species, Big Health recognizes the continuity of all life and the massively interconnected nature of health itself. When we talk about the health of people in habitat, it's not enough to look at isolated organisms, conditions or variables; we must include the continuous traffic between bodies, minds, environment and society.

In the early days of medicine, physicians could only focus on the health of individuals. Shamans, mystics and broad-minded doctors surely guessed at the health relationships that existed outside and beyond the body, but there was little hard evidence to make such a case. Today however, we have an enormous body of knowledge that proves without question that human health is tightly intertwined with other people, microorganisms, soil, plants, animals and the biosphere at large. Just as our sense of history has expanded by orders of magnitude over the last two centuries, so too has our understanding of health and disease.

This modern orientation towards Big Health is strikingly reminiscent of the holistic orientations described by so many indigenous cultures, from the Ju Wasi of the Kalahari to the aboriginals of Australia. Almost without exception, native peoples describe a comprehensive philosophy that includes mind, body, spirit, land, ancestors and tribe. In aboriginal cultures, all of these elements are essential to a complete human experience and to the health; it simply makes no sense to think of the body in isolation.

Today, we see a rapidly-growing body of scientific verification for many of these linkages. In fact, we are now seeing a powerful trend towards multi-disciplinary and trans-disciplinary studies that cross the circle from body to mind, land, tribe and spirit. There has been a proliferation of such academic alliances in recent decades—an effort to knit and weave previously isolated knowledge specialties into a more comprehensive view of the body and the world. Here's a brief list of such integrative disciplines:

- biopsychosocial medicine
- medical anthropology
- psychogeography
- sensory ecology
- cognitive ecology
- cognitive geography
- social endocrinology
- social neuroscience
- psychoneuroimmunology
- psychocultural studies
- social psychology
- body-centered psychotherapy
- evolutionary psychology
- evolutionary health and fitness

Taken individually, each of these disciplines is plenty fascinating and well worth exploring in its own right. But taken together, they demonstrate a powerful trend towards an integrated world view, a Big Health, Big Knowledge synthesis that promises to illuminate the myriad ways that our minds, bodies and spirits are connected to the social and living world.

CULTURE JAM

As we set out to explore the perplexing state of the human animal, it's inevitable that we'll be drawn into a discussion of origins. Where did modern disease and atrophy come from? What is the ultimate source of our physical discontent?

These are questions of causation, a study formally known as "etiology." The word is derived from the Greek *aitiologia*, or "giving a reason for." Few of us use this word in casual conversation, but in fact many of us love to talk etiology. We are naturally curious about disease and injury and we want to avoid becoming victims ourselves. And so we study, formally or informally, working the threads backwards from our various afflictions, always trying to get to the root. If we can identify the ultimate cause, maybe we can devise an antidote, or at least uncover a satisfying explanation that will set our minds at ease.

So what is the ultimate cause for today's lifestyle disease, our physical atrophy and malaise? The knee-jerk answers are familiar and by now, intensely boring. According to popular accounts, sedentary living, bad food choices, stress and toxins are the usual suspects. People eat too much, drink too much and sit on the couch too much. People just need to exercise more, start eating better and learn to relax, right?

This standard explanation is correct, but it's not nearly ultimate enough for our purposes. Yes, sedentary behavior and toxic food-like substances are important contributors to our condition, but these are matters of lifestyle and are often a matter of choice. And this begs a deeper question: why do people make the health choices that they do? Not because of some rational evaluation of costs and benefits; nobody I know reads the scientific literature before eating at the mini-mart or deciding to skip out on physical movement. Rather, we make lifestyle choices because of social contagion. We make poor health choices because we see others around us making similar choices. We are lifestyle mimics; we adopt destructive lifestyles because our friends, families and neighbors inspire us to do so. And in this sense, lifestyle diseases are the product of the culture that we live in.

If we follow the chain of causation backwards far enough, it soon becomes clear that culture has a lot to do with health and disease. It also becomes clear that, if we're going to get serious about health in the modern world, we're going to have to take our culture to task. We're going to have to get outside or beyond our immediate culture. In other words, our inquiry must be meta-cultural.

After all, if our culture is in fact the problem, it does little to remain at its own level. It makes little sense to seek health guidance from within the mindset that created the problem in the first place. As Einstein put it, "You can't solve a problem on the same level that created it."

FROM ME TO WE

As you'll soon discover, this book takes issue with the prevailing "me industry," especially as it appears in the world of pop health, fitness and fashion. In magazines, TV shows and other media, this industry relentlessly promotes the experience of the individual, completely without regard to community, tribe or habitat. Paradoxically, this orientation is proving to be increasingly destructive, not only to community and relationship with the world at large, but to the very individuals that the industry supposedly champions.

One look at the magazine rack is all it takes to get the picture. We see beautiful individual bodies on display in their Photoshopped glory: gorgeous, fantastic bodies, completely devoid of background, context, environment or habitat. These bodies are spectacular, but they lack a life-support system. They are wonderful, but doomed. Beautiful, but irrelevant.

The "me industry" is built on the misguided belief that the human body is a stand-alone organism and that health is all about individual function, performance and well-being. Before-and-after pictures look like evidence of success, but this is a temporary illusion at best. By isolating individuals from their environment, the "me industry" actually sabotages the health that it claims to promote. Even in the world of holistic health—a practice dedicated to mind, body and spirit—attention is typically focused on the individual's mind, the individual's body and individual's spirit. It's all about *me* or it's all about *you*, but it's never about *us*.

In fact, things that happen outside of our skin have powerful effects on the state of our bodies and lives. Our health waxes and wanes with changes in climate, flora, fauna, soils and habitat. We are deeply embedded in our biological and social worlds; isolation is a dangerous illusion.

By shifting the focus from "me" to "we," we can actually improve the health of our bodies and in turn, the world at large. Our task is to challenge the culture that produces today's body-destructive lifestyle and create a new, life-promoting alternative. And so, this book is intentionally subversive and counter-cultural. It points to the folly of the "me industry" and when possible, exposes its oversights and extremity. It recommends that we throw off the myopic focus on single individuals and concentrate instead on relationships, systems and processes. It takes on convention, assumptions and tradition. So be forewarned: This is not a safe book.

WHAT'S IN IT FOR US?

Since books are purchased and read by individuals, it seems sensible to inquire as to how an individual might benefit from reading this one. But in light of what we now know about the human body, the question seems paradoxical and gets us started off on the wrong foot. It asks, in effect, "How will taking the focus off *me* benefit *me*?"

So we begin with a caution: Yes, you'll find ideas here that will improve the condition of your body. You may even pick up some clues that will help you look and feel better. You just might discover ways to improve your performance, recover from injury faster or live a little bit longer. If you take these suggestions to heart, you'll probably lose a few pounds, gain some muscular strength and enjoy a renewed sense of vitality.

But these are inadvertent, tangential benefits. The real goal is to explore the way we create our bodies in relationship to culture and our world. It's all about creating a virtuous circle: If we can take a few steps towards creating a healthier *we*, we're likely to create a healthier *me* as well. Along the way, you'll enjoy some tangible benefits to body and health. In the process, you'll

- create a more meaningful sense of health
- increase your physical happiness
- expand your sense of possibility in human movement
- align your quest for health with the pressing issues of the modern world
- broaden and extend your vision of what it means to be healthy
- contribute to a healthier habitat

It's all about creating cycles of positive causality, life-affirming ideas, memes and behaviors that feed back on themselves to generate even more of their original essence. Do some vigorous movement for a few weeks and you'll enjoy an elevated mood and improved cognitive function. In turn, your elevated outlook will give you the incentive to pursue more ambitious challenges. You'll not only feel better, but you'll want to get out explore and engage the world.

This process naturally ripples outward to broader levels of society, culture and environment: Healthier people tend to create healthier organizations. They are less depressed, less hostile and make better decisions. They are more ambiguity-tolerant and stress-resistant. This adds up to improved social and organizational performance, which in turn brings more benefits to everyone involved.

INTO THE BUSH

So off we go on our walkabout, into this terrain of essays and commentary. Our journey will take us deep into a bushy habitat of bodies, health, physical training, culture and lifeways. As with any journey into the bush, the trail will branch off several directions, wandering its way into a mosaic landscape of hills, mountains, river valleys, marshes and vistas.

As you read these essays, don't expect a linear sidewalk with bright lines, mileage markers and GPS coordinates. This book is not a linear narrative. Rather, it's the creation of a wild animal mind coming to grips with its predicament. You won't find curbs, escalators or handrails on your path; you won't be able to download a map onto your smartphone or get real-time position reports of your progress. Instead, expect to find a good many roots and rocks, even some downed trees, snowfields and cliffs. Don't be surprised if the trail takes you in some new and surprising directions.

And this is precisely the point. Natural travel is always a negotiation between body and terrain. So use your senses and stay alert for opportunity. Follow the path as you see it, but craft your own story and meaning as you go. Get your body involved in the process of observation and understanding. Pay attention to the lay of the land and you'll find your way.

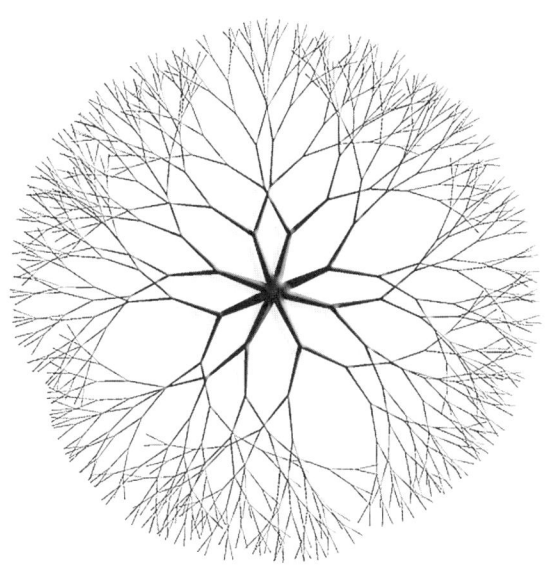

BODY TALK

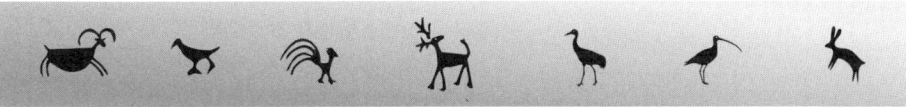

Change Your Body, Change the World

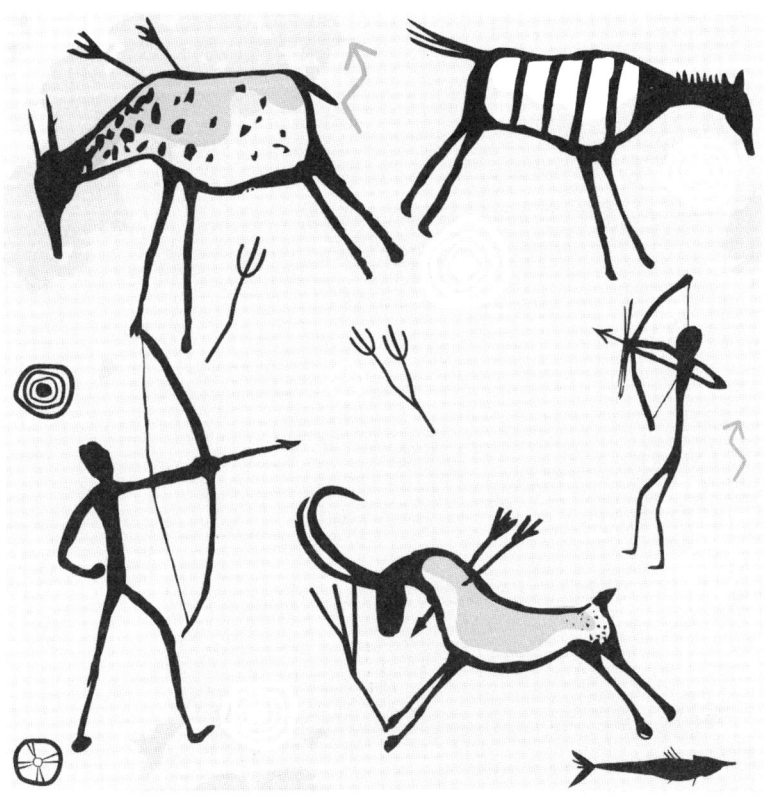

PRIMATE'S PREDICAMENT

> The deviation of man from the state in which he was originally placed by nature seems to have proved to him a prolific source of diseases.
>
> Edward Jenner

> He who conceals his disease cannot expect to be cured.
>
> Ethiopian Proverb

So what's the state of the animal in the modern world? Is he living large or just getting by? Is his body happy and powerful or is he suffering in a state of injury and disease?

Opinions vary, but it's starting to look like a "good news, bad news" situation. The good news is that lifespans are up. People are living longer than ever before in recent history and for many, the quality of life is comfortable, even wonderful. If you have the resources, modern life is not only easy, it's filled to bursting with opportunities for experience, learning and growth. If you have the resources, you can get excellent food year-round, expert medical care and access to education that is absolutely mind-blowing. If you have the resources, you can live a life of incredibly robust health and vitality.

But sadly, there's also a lot of bad news for the human body and for human life as a whole. For all the increases in lifespan and life quality for the affluent, too many of our bodies are suffering. A quick look around our public spaces tells the story: an enormous percentage of us are obese and for all practical purposes, physically disempowered—unable to run, jump, play or enjoy our native physicality. Surveys consistently reveal high levels of body dissatisfaction, even among people who are otherwise healthy. The paradox is striking: the human body, living in the midst of the greatest health opportunities in human history, has become weak, dysfunctional and physically illiterate.

By almost any definition or measure, serious disease is rampant. Obesity, heart disease, diabetes, metabolic syndrome, depression, neurological disorders and cancer are not just widespread; they are quickly becoming the norm. Only a few thousand years ago, humans were robust, vibrant, highly functional wild animals, but today, we are chronically diseased and in nearly constant need of pharmaceuticals, surgery and other heroic treatments.

Actual physical disease is obviously a major problem, but it's just the tip of an enormous psychosocial iceberg. Unhappy bodies pull our spirits down into vicious cycles of decreasing vitality, weakened immunity, poor decision-making and further physical unhappiness. Even worse, ill health ripples throughout society; as lifestyle disease becomes widespread, ever more people succumb to its pull.

Of course, humans have always faced injury and disease. Physical pain and injury have long been part of the human experience, indeed part of the experience of all animals. Throughout the grand scope of human history, our species has always faced physical and health challenges, no doubt going back to our history as tree-dwelling primates. But what we're seeing in the world today is something different, unique and profoundly disturbing. If present trends continue, *Homo sapiens* is soon to become a chronically diseased animal.

ACT ONE: THE PALEO

The history of human disease plays out in three main acts. To get the picture, let's begin by going back a million years or so to the world of our primal, hominid ancestors. In this Paleo world, insults to the hominid body were physically dramatic, sometimes acute. Infant mortality was probably high, exposure and dehydration were not uncommon. Hunters and gatherers probably suffered bruises, sprained ankles and lacerations, not to mention the dramatically life-threatening challenges of snakebites and predation.

Nevertheless, primal peoples enjoyed generally robust health and high levels of physical capability. Infectious disease epidemics were either rare or unknown. When people live in small, widely dispersed tribal bands, virulent microorganisms simply do not have the opportunity to circulate and multiply. If pathogens take hold in a small tribe, they might well very well wreak havoc, but the tribe would either die out or disperse, leaving other tribes unaffected.

ACT TWO: THE AGE OF INFECTION

As humankind entered the age of agriculture around 10,000 years ago, patterns of physical affliction changed dramatically; we began to experience a radically new threat of infectious disease. Increasingly crowded conditions, poor sanitation and active commerce between regions combined to produce drastic increases in infectious disease mortality.

A quick Wikipedia search reminds us just how lethal microorganisms can be:

> The Black Death of 1347–1352 killed 25 million in Europe. (25–50% of the populations of Europe, Asia, and Africa).
>
> The introduction of smallpox, measles, and typhus to Central and South America by European explorers during the 15th and 16th centuries caused pandemics among the native inhabitants. Between 1518 and 1568 the population of Mexico fell from 20 million to 3 million.
>
> Smallpox killed an estimated 60 million Europeans during the 18th century. (approximately 400,000 per year)
>
> In the 19th century, tuberculosis killed an estimated one-quarter of the adult population of Europe.
>
> The Influenza Pandemic of 1918 killed 25-50 million people (about 2% of the world population).

ACT THREE: LIFESTYLE DISEASE

Given the sheer carnage inflicted by microorganisms, it's not surprising that the survivors of infectious disease stepped up to create a range of countermeasures. We developed vaccines, sanitation and education to keep most of infectious epidemics at bay. Today, the threat of infectious disease continues to linger in the background, but it tends to be far removed from day-to-day consciousness, especially in the affluent West. Few of us worry about smallpox, polio or the plague anymore.

What's different today is the rapid increase in "lifestyle disease," afflictions that have nothing to do with microorganisms: obesity, heart disease, diabetes, metabolic syndrome, depression and, to some extent, cancer. These are the so-called "non-communicable diseases" or NCDs.

The death toll from these largely preventable conditions is enormous and growing. According to the World Health Organization website more than 35 million people died of NCDs in 2005 — this represented 60% of all deaths worldwide.

This figure is appalling of course, but it doesn't begin to reveal the true extent of the catastrophe: for every person who dies of obesity, diabetes or heart disease, thousands more live lives of diminished movement, vitality and joy.

PALEO BODIES IN AN ALIEN ENVIRONMENT

To get to the root of our predicament, we need to understand that we are, in a very real sense, living out of context. Our bodies have a long history of evolution and adaptation in natural environments, but today we live in an entirely different world.

Many anthropologists, biologists and physicians have made this observation, but most individuals in our society have yet to feel the true extent of the mismatch. Without an appreciation for our deep physical history, many of are duped by the modern world. We adapt quickly to the circumstances of our birth and may even come to believe that things have always been the way they are today—that a world of cars, couches, concrete and computers is normal and natural.

But when we take the long view of human history, we begin to realize that our modern industrialized world is neither normal nor natural. Today's challenges are unique and we are ill-prepared to deal with them. Our aboriginal impulses, once a powerful force for survival and health, have now become threats to our vitality and our well-being.

To really understand the depth of mismatch between our physical heritage and the modern environment, it's essential that we imagine human prehistory in detail. When we do, we begin to realize that until quite recently, we were highly intelligent wild animals living in natural outdoor environments. We lived outdoors all day, every day, squeezing out a living from the land.

Thousands of generations of evolution sculpted our bodies and brains to fit the conditions of the natural world. In fact, every detail of our anatomy and physiology is the way it is because it helped us to survive on the semi-wooded grasslands of East Africa. In our essential form, our bodies are all aboriginal, all African, all indigenous. Our bodies and brains are run by legacy programming from this not-so-distant past. And now we find ourselves living in a world of radically different character: an alien environment.

WELCOME TO YOUR ALIEN WORLD

The modern environment is alien to the human body in many ways. Most conspicuously, it is clear that we now live in an alien kinetic environment. We are no longer required to move our bodies in any significant or sustained way. Walking, once the gold standard of human movement, is now almost entirely optional for the modern American. The hunter-gatherer daily average, often estimated at 5-10 miles, now seems like an outrageous hardship to most.

It's also clear that we live in an alien nutritional environment. Only a few thousand years ago, all food was wild, organic, local and unprocessed. Today, almost everything we find on our grocery store shelves is processed, refined and trucked in from some remote location. No longer do we eat real food obtained by our own hands or by those of a tribe member; we eat "edible food-like substances" that are completely divorced from the land. Not only do we eat immense quantities of food, we have no idea where most of it comes from.

Our sensory environment is also alien. Because we no longer walk the land, our vision is distorted. Instead of scanning a three-dimensional world for danger and opportunity, we fix our vision on a single point in space, either a computer cursor or the bumper of the car in front of us. Hearing is under constant assault by noise almost everywhere we go. Skin is protected from all manner of heat, cold, sun and contact. Indoor textures have been smoothed down to featureless, plastic monotony. Natural odors are masked by (often toxic) airborne chemicals wafting through our homes, cars and workplaces. And our feet, bound up in shoes almost from the day of our birth, no longer feel the tones of the earth.

Our circadian experience is profoundly alien as well. We no longer pay much attention to the master physiological regulator, sunlight. Instead, we substitute a weak, artificial imposter that plays havoc with every metabolic process in our bodies. Distorted light-dark cycles, jet lag and shift work punish our bodies in ways never before experienced by human beings.

We also live in an alien choice environment. All across our experience, from the mall to the office to the household, we face an explosion of options. There are thousands of decisions to be made each day in matters of commerce, education, finance, technology, administration and medicine. We have more tools, more methods, more information and more complexity than ever before. This crushing load of choice is profoundly abnormal and extremely stressful.

To make matters even more challenging, we now live in an alien social environment. By nature a hyper-social tribal animal, we have lived the vast majority of our time on earth in small bands of 20 to 100 people. Our social brains, awareness and sensitivities are all wired for small group living. But today, our "tribes" are either very small or extremely large by comparison. We suffer from loneliness or are overwhelmed with social stimulation, or both. Workplace "tribes" are organized around corporate priorities, not human social needs. Online networks bring us into patterns of relationship that are entirely without precedent.

INVERTED PERSPECTIVE

Depending on your childhood experience, this claim that the modern world is "alien" will seem either obvious or preposterous. If you've grown up in the outback of Australia or the rural backwoods of North America, the wild outdoors is your reference point for how the world looks and feels; the natural outdoor world is "normal" and the shopping mall is "alien." But if you are one of the millions who have grown up in a shopping mall-cubicle-SUV world, you may come to the opposite, unconscious conclusion that the mall is "normal" and the natural outdoor world is "alien."

Of all the tragedies of the modern world, this is perhaps the most disturbing and dangerous. Not only have we positioned ourselves outside the source of life, many of us now feel that nature itself is alien. Too many of us, especially young people, now feel comfortable only in insulated, artificial circumstances and are reluctant to expose their bodies to the very things that would promote health and happiness. Our native habitat of land, water, plants and animals now feels like an unfamiliar and hostile world: nature now feels like other. Woody Allen spoke for far too many of us when he described his relationship with the natural world: "Nature and I are two."

A PARADOXICAL PREDICAMENT

Like it or not, we live in a world that is profoundly dangerous to our bodies, minds, spirits and our future. This statement, of course, sounds odd to many modern ears. After all, unless you live in a war zone, today's world doesn't look or feel particularly hostile. On the contrary, we see ample evidence of body-friendly conditions everywhere we look. Modern buildings keep us warm, dry and cool. Modern clothing keeps us clean and comfortable. Modern vehicles take us where we want to go. Our modern food industry delivers ample calories to us virtually on demand.

Yet this is precisely the problem. The hostility of the modern world doesn't come in the form of extreme heat and cold, lightning strikes or predator attacks. Rather, it comes in the form of excess ease, insulation and affluence. The modern environment is hostile precisely because it's too comfortable. It's hostile because it no longer challenges our bodies to sweat, strain or struggle. And without physical challenge, our tissue quickly breaks down. Physiology and psychology begin to drift, unable to find a relationship with the world at large. Without challenge, the organism loses focus and becomes susceptible to disease and dysfunction.

This is one of the most striking ironies of modern civilization: by engineering our environment to take care of our every physical need and desire, we have simultaneously disempowered ourselves and brought disease upon our bodies. What makes our modern epidemic so perplexing is that it's self-inflicted—not consciously, intentionally or masochistically, but engineered by our own hands nonetheless. This makes our challenge doubly difficult. Not only do we have to deal with the actual physiology and biochemistry of the diseases themselves, we also have to alter the strategies, institutions, behaviors and values that brought us to this point. Far more is required than simply healing individual people; we have to transform the culture that brought us here.

ON THE BRINK

Unfortunately, we are completely unprepared to meet this challenge. We lack knowledge, ideas and orientation. In this sense, we are like peasants of the Middle Ages, standing in our fields and villages, watching in horror as infectious disease ravages our communities. People are sick and dying in vast numbers all around us, but we feel powerless to save them.

The magnitude and severity of today's lifestyle diseases may not be as dramatic or lethal as the Black Plague, but they are deadly serious all the same and like our peasant ancestors, we are woefully unprepared to deal. The naked fact of public health in the modern world is that, for all our advice and pronouncements about what needs to be done to support human health, we really have no experience to work with. We are at the zero point in this epidemic and it's time for us to learn fast.

A CALL FOR CREATIVE DISRUPTION

As we stand on the brink of this unique and disturbing public health catastrophe, one thing becomes obvious: our situation calls for radical and disruptive creativity. Given the paradoxical and urgent qualities of this modern day lifestyle plague, we cannot hope to make progress with conventional, culture-as-usual solutions.

The body, when left to its own devices, will commit a form of slow-motion suicide. Our paradoxical challenge is to save the human body from its Paleolithic impulses and inclinations. Those things that feel easy—sloth and high-calorie foods most notoriously—lead towards disease. To save the body, we need to do things that may feel wrong, things that feel challenging and uncomfortable.

Conventional solutions merely rearrange the deck chairs on our public health Titanic. It's not enough to say that people need to exercise more and eat less. And it's clearly not enough to seek a techno-pharmaceutical solution to every physical and psychological ailment.

What we need is disruptive creativity and paradoxical prescriptions. In other words, we need some crazy-sounding ideas, ideas that run counter to our conventional impulses and institutions. Instead of seeking ever more efficient ways to make our lives easier, we need to find creative and interesting ways to make our lives harder, in some cases much harder. We need to find ways to reintroduce meaningful and sustained physical challenge into modern life. We need more exposure to the natural world: more heat and cold, more sweat and shivering, more contact with dirt, plants and animals, more scrapes and bruises, more heavy loads and long days. And above all, more physical risk. This means going against the grain of hundreds of years of Western industrial culture and commerce.

Naturally, this proposal will be a hard sell and opposition will be instantaneous. We are heavily invested in physical comfort, ease and insulation from the natural world. Entire industries are dedicated to taking physical effort out of human life. People will protest and claim their right physical apathy, but the challenge remains and it's time to step up, both literally and symbolically. It's time to expose our bodies to the natural world and walk the path of physical hardship. The body needs some tough physical love.

ESCAPE FROM THE CAVE

As we ponder the state of the modern human animal and our increasing isolation from the natural world, we're reminded of Plato's famous Allegory of the Cave. In *The Republic,* Plato imagined a group of people chained in a cave all of their lives, facing a blank wall. These people watched shadows projected on the wall by a fire, and began to ascribe forms to them. According to Plato, the shadows are as close as the prisoners get to seeing reality.

The allegory is a spot-on description for the alienated and denatured consciousness of the modern world. The cave, of course, is the insulated world of the shopping mall, airport, cubicle and SUV. Young people grow up in this cave and come to perceive it as normal. They watch transfixed as the digital shadows flicker on the walls of these caves, oblivious to the wider world outside.

Because we are a highly adaptable species, we are good at adjusting to life in the cave and we may even come to see it as "normal." But ultimately the cave is dangerous to our health and even our sanity. Our minds and bodies can adapt to almost anything, but the cave insulates us from the very forces that sustain our vitality.

To preserve our health, vitality and happiness, it is essential that we get out of the cave and integrate ourselves back into the natural, outside world. This suggests a new, more expansive role for today's trainers, leaders, teachers, therapists, coaches and senseis. For Plato, the philosopher was like a prisoner who is freed from the cave and who understands that the shadows on the wall do not represent reality. The philosopher's purpose is to show the path out of the cave, back to the land, back to habitat and back to vitality and health.

Today's trainers, leaders, teachers, therapists and coaches can take a similar role. We may be in the business of teaching specific skills, knowledge and ideas, but beyond this content lies a larger and more compelling purpose: showing people the way out of the cave, into the natural physical and living world. Open the door for people to reconnect with the forces, qualities and elements that give our bodies life. Let's lead by example and show our students what "normal" really is.

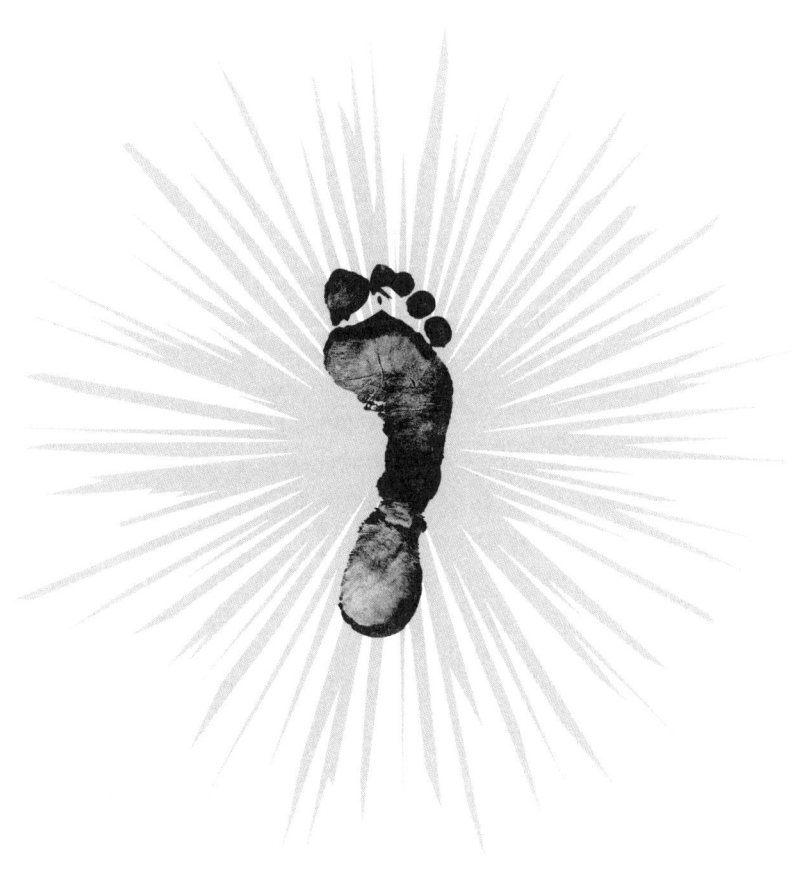

Change Your Body, Change the World

THE FIRST THING THAT HAPPENS

Tell me to what you pay attention and I will tell you who you are.

Jose Ortega y Gasset

The moment one gives close attention to any thing, even a blade of grass, it becomes a mysterious, awesome, indescribably magnificent world in itself.

Henry Miller

The highest ecstasy is the attention at its fullest.

Simone Weil

If you ever have the chance to hike the mountains and river valleys of the Olympic Peninsula in the Pacific Northwest, you just might run into a charismatic movement teacher called the Barefoot Sensei. The Sensei has been barefooting for almost 20 years and is a passionate advocate for the practice. Not only does he walk the walk, he also spreads the word wherever he goes, talking the talk in coffee shops, bookstores, campgrounds and parks. He tells a story of personal transformation through barefooting and teaches people how to get back into their bodies. People call him the Barefoot Sensei for good reason: he's discovered an inspiring and practical way to reinvigorate human life experience, starting with the foot.

When the Sensei gives presentations on the virtues of barefooting, he often begins with a simple question:

"What's the first thing that happens when you take your shoes off?"

His students grope for an answer, searching their memory banks for the last time they actually went barefoot, suspicious that this might be some sort of trick question. But before they can get their words in order, Sensei answers for them:

"You start paying attention!"

Some listeners find this amusing or trivial, but it's actually quite profound, something that will immediately become obvious to anyone who actually spends time outdoors in bare feet. When you kick your shoes off, it doesn't take long for the instinct for foot preservation to kick in. There's something about naked, vulnerable feet that brings the bodymind into sharp focus. Stop paying attention for a few moments and you'll see, or rather feel, what Sensei is getting at. Just try thinking about your relationship troubles, your floundering career or your to-do list while you're running barefoot down a rocky trail; you'll get a reminder soon enough. Stub your toe on a rock and your mind will return to the present moment in an instant.

THE BAREFOOT MEDITATION

In a world plagued by distraction and over-stimulation, we've invented a vast range of techniques for focusing our minds. We have a hundred forms of meditation and mental training. We have CDs, retreat centers and mantras. We have computer programs and pharmaceuticals.

But aren't we forgetting something fundamental? Aren't we forgetting about our "lower education?" Human ancestors didn't need supplemental meditative practices; they were focusing and refocusing their attention throughout the course of every barefoot day. As soon as they rose each morning and took their first steps, awareness kicked in and brought attention to the challenge of moving through habitat. A hunter-gatherer might try to multi-task or split her attention, but rocks, sticks, roots and holes would quickly bring the mind back to the here and now. No esoteric training techniques required.

In essence, barefooting is a 6 million year-old meditation and a powerful one at that, especially if you travel on diverse terrain, moving with intent and purpose. Every step demands focus and concentration. Every step demands a neuromuscular calculation. Every step demands grace, precision and adjustment.

So might it not make sense to use barefooting as a path to increased powers of concentration? It's simple and it's free. Just get out of your shoes and start footing the path. Your mind will follow in short order. Your sensitive feet will lead the rest of your body and mind into the present moment. No schooling or training required. It's just you, your bare feet and the earth.

MODERNITY

The Barefoot Sensei likes his koan, but he might very well cast his question in reverse: "What's the first thing that happens when you put your shoes *on*?"

The answer, grasshopper, is simple: "You *stop* paying attention."

This, in short, is the story of human attention in modern civilization. The transition took a few centuries, but the effects of footwear and similar forms of insulation have been disastrous. As our footwear "improved," we started paying less attention to the world around us. We started paying less attention to terrain and texture of course, but also to the natural world in general.

Modernity itself might even be described as a process of decreasing physical sensitivity, mediated by shoes, clothing, cars and dwellings. The process began innocently enough, with simple and sensible measures to comfort and protect our bodies and our skin. A pair of sandals reduces abrasion, allows us to move faster and opens up some new terrain.

So far, so good. But if a little insulation is good, more must be better, so on we went to thicker soles, thicker clothes and tighter dwellings. Innovation drove this trend forward, always covering, protecting and insulating the body. After a few thousand years, we've come to a tipping point of rapidly diminishing returns. Suddenly, our insulating technologies begin to compromise the quality of our lives and separate us from the very source of life.

Footwear might well be described as a "gateway technology" that put us on the slippery slope to environmental amnesia. Today we move through the world as if armored in psychophysical Kevlar. We've lost our sense of physical vulnerability and consequently, there's not much point in paying attention. Ultimately, this process becomes pathological. When the body is massively insulated and protected, sensation goes dormant through disuse and our bodies go blind. Tragically, we become desensitized precisely at a time when we should be paying more attention than ever to the world around us.

BAREFOOT ZANSHIN

In the world of martial art, teachers often encourage their students to sharpen their powers of attention. Specifically, they promote the exercise of *zanshin*. There are several interpretations of this word, but in essence, *zanshin* refers to focused concentration and awareness. In my dojo, our sensei emphasized *zanshin* by reminding us to "always train as if you're facing a live blade." We even practiced with real swords on occasion to focus our training and sharpen our attention.

This method is incredibly effective, of course. When there's a naked samurai sword in the room, everyone knows it and everyone pays close attention; you can literally feel the threat of the blade as soon as it's drawn from the scabbard. Suddenly, people are focused and alert. Bodies are ready for movement, right here, right now.

The sword is a dramatic stimulus for heightened attention, but we can get a similar result simply by taking our shoes off in the outdoors. A smooth, carpeted studio or dojo is not ideal for this purpose; what we really need is a natural habitat with roots, rocks, holes and other hazards. Once we step out with naked feet into this kind of world, we create a sense of *barefoot zanshin*.

The effect is immediate and profoundly psychophysical. Sharp rocks and sticks are just as effective as a samurai sword in bringing our attention into the present moment. Danger focuses the mind. Risk stimulates the sympathetic nervous system and generates a slight elevation in the stress hormone cortisol. This hormone, in small doses, has a powerful effect on consciousness and memory formation. It won't produce a full-blown fight-flight response, but it's enough to sharpen attention.

SERIOUS, BUT NOT LETHAL

For beginners, the very idea of outdoor barefooting seems extreme and brings up a lot of apprehension. "What if I step on a sharp rock?" is the common concern.

The solution lies in attention. Stay in the moment and step mindfully; keep looking, keep adjusting, keep working your eye-foot coordination. This is the nature of the practice.

Of course, there will be miscalculations. You will almost certainly step on sharp rocks from time to time, but you will also discover that your body is much smarter than you give it credit for. Our legs and spinal cords are wired with reflexes that prevent catastrophe. When you step on a sharp stone, sensory information will flash up your legs, synapse with neurons in your spinal cord and instantly inhibit the appropriate motor commands, causing you to unweight the leg in question, thus preserving the skin on the underside of your foot.

This process is unconscious, blindingly fast and completely reliable. It works wonders. In my barefoot hikes, I've miscalculated many times, stepping on stones that might well have lacerated or punctured the soles of my feet. But aside from occasional scrapes, I never suffer injury. Almost by magic, my body compensates for dangerous footing. I stumble a bit and continue on, none the worse for wear. The foot survives.

So, while outdoor barefooting remains a serious practice, it is less dangerous than most people realize. Give your body a chance and it will figure out what to do.

FLOW

Barefoot *zanshin* shares a good many characteristics with the flow state described by Mihaly Csikszentmihalyi in his landmark book *Flow: The Psychology of Optimal Experience*. Flow is the mental state in which a person is fully immersed in what he or she is doing. It's characterized by a feeling of energized focus and full absorption.

Csikszentmihalyi's description of flow applies perfectly to the barefoot experience, especially when we're really getting into it, running across diverse, natural terrain. In the process, we experience the classic elements of flow:

- concentrating and focusing
- a loss of self-consciousness, the merging of action and awareness
- a distorted sense of time
- balance between ability level and challenge
- a sense of personal control
- a sense that the activity is intrinsically rewarding, so there is an effortlessness of action.
- the focus of awareness is narrowed down to the activity itself.

Call it *zanshin* or call it "flow," it makes little difference; barefooting is all about the here and now.

ENVIRONMENTAL ZANSHIN

When we practice barefooting regularly, our attention will eventually grow into a wider "environmental zanshin," an expansive, but highly focused awareness of all things local and immediate. The attention we enjoy in bare feet naturally extends outward to other environmental qualities. Not only does our foot sensitivity increase, we also experience a general sharpening of the senses. It's not just the shape of the rocks and sticks on the trail itself that grabs our attention. We also become increasingly aware of air temperature, changes in light, odor, movement, wind and sound. Naked feet inspire us to gather information in every direction. The vulnerable body wants to know all that it can.

This form of attention is immensely rewarding and is extremely relevant to our modern predicament. As technology becomes ever more refined, we have come to rely on external sensors to tell us about the state of our world. In effect, we have out-sourced much of our sensation to external instruments that tell us about temperature, light, moisture and other environmental qualities. Our bodies are no longer involved in the basic challenge of knowing the world. This leaves us with a creeping sense of psychological unease.

For all creatures, sensory engagement with the world is vital to health, performance and a sense of well-being; we desperately need a sensory conversation with the world. This is vital, not just to our personal health as individuals, but also to our ability to preserve what's left of the natural world. To value and protect a thing, we must know it in our bodies and in our flesh. So find yourself a path, take off your shoes and feel the earth. Not only will your body become smarter, you'll find yourself rejoicing in new-found sensations of delight.

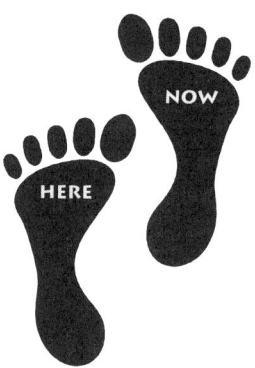

NO BODY IS AN ISLAND

Your self does not end where your flesh ends, but suffuses and blends with the world, including other beings.

> Sandra Blakeslee and Matthew Blakeslee
> *The Body Has a Mind of Its Own*

When we try to pick out anything by itself, we find it hitched to everything else in the Universe.

> John Muir
> *My First Summer in the Sierra (1911)*

No man is an island, entire of itself...

> John Donne 1572–1631
> *Meditation XVII*

When we take a quick look at the human body, the nature of the thing seems perfectly obvious. It looks like a stand-alone object, an individual organism, bounded by skin. It's got a form that's easy to recognize and that form remains stable, with minor changes, for decades. There are inflows and outflows of solids, liquids and gasses, but otherwise it's basically a system unto itself—a unit.

The singular appearance of the human body is confirmed—so it would seem—by our subjective life experience. Just as we look like individuals, we also feel like individuals. There's a "me" and a "you" and unless we are lovers in the throes of passion, we remain as singular, individual bodies for the better part of our lives. I am one and you are one and the environment is "out there."

Our perception of physical singularity also seems validated by the doctor's anatomy chart. The body is right there on the wall, laid out in crisp graphic detail. The skin has disappeared of course, but there can be no question: the body stands alone, unconnected to any other force, form or process. Popular magazine covers give us the same impression except that now the skin and form are Photoshopped to sexually-idealized perfection; there's no background, no context and no life support.

HEALTH IS EXTRASOMATIC

Our perception of the human body as a singular, isolated unit, strong as it may happen to be, is actually an illusion and a dangerous one at that. While we can and do function as individuals, we are massively interconnected with the biological and social world around us. In fact, it's not altogether clear where the human body begins and ends.

This is one of the most revolutionary discoveries in the world of medicine and public health of the last few decades. Findings in the fields of molecular biology, epidemiology, public health, stress medicine and social neuroscience have revealed without question that our health is profoundly influenced by extrasomatic forces that operate beyond the body.

This means that, for all practical purposes, our bodies are bigger than they look and bigger than they feel. There are myriad processes beyond the reach of our fingertips, forces that profoundly affect the functioning of our organs and our tissue. Our bodies are shaped in large measure by things that happen remotely, both in space and time.

Mystics and shamans have suspected as much for thousands of years, but now we are beginning to see our extrasomatic relationships in more concrete, scientific terms. The skin is not a barrier to the world, merely a transitional membrane. Our bodies may appear to us as isolated, stand-alone organisms, but in fact, they are in constant relationship, communication and interchange with other people and processes, many of which affect our health in surprising and profound ways.

WE ARE EMBEDDED

One of the most striking challenges to the isolationist view of the body is the discovery of vast populations of non-human organisms both in and around us. Latest estimates have it that only one in ten cells in and around the human body are actually human tissue cells. We are literally awash in other organisms, mostly bacteria. Those organisms are living, metabolizing, discharging wastes, multiplying and dying in great numbers, every second of every day.

You can wash your skin all you like and detoxify your gut for weeks on end, but you can never change this fundamental fact of human existence. In fact, if we were to somehow kill all of the "not-I" organisms in and around our bodies, we would die in short order; these microbes are absolutely essential to the proper functioning of our immune and digestive systems. Like it or not, you can never be a single organism—more properly, you are an ecosystem with legs.

We also see a profound interconnection between human bodies in our shared immunity against pathogenic (disease-causing) microbes. Remember the last time someone coughed in a crowded room or sneezed in an elevator? We know, almost without being told, that germs are spreading and threatening our health. But there's a wider meaning here that goes beyond the threat to individual health. That is, humans are constantly exchanging microorganisms with one another and in this sense, our personal immune systems are actually parts of a much larger, networked meta-system. My health depends not just on my behavior and my relationship to the microbial world, but on the success of other immune systems in my neighborhood, community and workplace. If my neighbor's immunity is compromised for some reason, the microbial challenge eventually gets shifted onto everyone else. Like it or not, we are all participating in the same struggle against the microbial world; immunity is a community enterprise.

On a macro level, we see a massive interconnection between individual human bodies and habitat. We are constantly engaged in a chemical and energy exchange with surrounding plants, animals, air and soil. Everything that we eat, drink and breathe is touched and transformed by other organisms around us. And yet, in an age of industrial agriculture, we forget this simple fact. When farms and factories are hundreds or thousands of miles away, we develop a delusion of individual autonomy and forget our connection to the rest of life.

In his book *Does it Matter?* Alan Watts reminded us that our life support comes from both within and without:

> ...civilized human beings are alarmingly ignorant of the fact that they are continuous with their natural surroundings. It is as necessary to have air, water, plants, insects, birds, fish

and mammals as it is to have brains, hearts, lungs and stomachs. The former are our external organs in the same way the latter are our internal organs.

SOCIAL AND CULTURAL CONTAGION

Ecological interdependence is just the beginning. Social and cultural forces are enormously influential in shaping individual health. Meaning and emotion flow between people constantly, even when no words are exchanged. Odors of fear and pleasure waft through the air and inform us—unconsciously—of prevailing emotional states. Posture and proximity allow us to touch one another's bodies without actually doing so. If I stand near you and move my body in a certain way, I can affect your hormone levels, your stress response and your cognition. Meaning flows in both directions, with bodies in constant conversation.

Emotions are not just experienced by individuals, but shared, unconsciously and unintentionally, across social groups. This is most powerful in real-time, face-to-face encounters as our mirror neuron systems read the emotional content of other bodies. The simple act of watching another person move affects how we feel, what we think and how we behave. In this way, emotion ripples and cascades through social systems, affecting the health of everyone in the process. In a very real way, we actually create one another's bodies and life experience.

POPULATION LEVEL

The interconnection between human bodies becomes even more apparent when we look at health and disease across large populations. In his book *The Status Syndrome*, epidemiologist Michael Marmot compiled thirty years of evidence demonstrating the crucial importance of social rank in health. His conclusion is that "Health follows a social gradient."

Marmot found that social inequalities are powerful determinants of health: "Wherever we are in the social hierarchy, our health is likely to be better than those below us and worse than those above us." This holds true, not just for one particular kind of illness, but for all forms of human affliction. "Being low in the hierarchy means a greater susceptibility to just about every disease that's going."

Marmot spent almost three decades studying the health of British civil servants, all classified according to their rank in the occupational hierarchy. The findings showed a dramatic gradient in mortality for most major causes of death: disease of the cardiovascular, renal, gastrointestinal, and respiratory systems, most cancers, accidental deaths and violent deaths. His conclusion was that "subtle differences in social ranking can lead to dramatic differences in health."

Michael Marmot's findings are echoed by findings of The Equality Trust, a UK non-profit organization. Their researchers compared the health of people in low and high-equality societies, revealing a consistent pattern: people in high-equality societies tend to be healthier. According to their website, there are now over 170 studies of income inequality in relation to various aspects of health. Life expectancy, infant mortality, low birth weight and self-rated health have repeatedly been shown to be worse in more unequal societies.

Research carried out since the early 1990s shows that many of the most pressing health and social problems are worse in more unequal societies. Societies with bigger income differences between rich and poor seem to suffer more of a wide range of health and social dysfunctions. (See *The Spirit Level: Why More Equal Societies Almost Always do Better* by Richard Wilkinson and Kate Pickett.)

IT'S ALL CONTAGIOUS

Health, we're now beginning to realize, is far more multi-dimensional than previously imagined. In fact, our bodies are part of an immensely complex, interconnected and chaotic system. This is not just poetic language—when an environmental butterfly flaps its wings on the other side of the planet, everyone's body is affected. Winds carry topsoil, dust, seeds and pathogens around the world. Pharmaceuticals pass through animal bodies and into the water supply where they are absorbed by other organisms. Fertilizers, pesticides and herbicides filter into rivers, lakes and aquifers. Plastic by-products find their way into our bodies, disrupting vital endocrine systems. Ultimately, our embedded bodies experience the ripples of energy and substances that course through the living world.

The discoveries of ecology and epidemiology are forcing us into drastic re-evaluations of some basic medical assumptions. For the last half century, we have divided human disease into two distinct categories: infectious diseases caused by pathogens such as bacteria and viruses, and non-infectious diseases caused by "lifestyle factors." But now it's starting to look like things are a lot more complicated. The problem is that the so-called "non-communicable" or "lifestyle" diseases may in fact be spread through social networks, influence and mimicked behavior. To say that heart disease, diabetes and obesity are matters of "lifestyle" misses the point because lifestyle itself is highly contagious. Lifestyle doesn't infect people the same way that smallpox does, but there is no longer any question of social and cultural contagion. An enormous percentage of our health and disease is "catching," in way or another.

NO HEALTH ISLANDS

Given what we now know about the tight interconnection of human health and the surrounding world, we are forced to ask some hard questions: Is it even possible to be healthy in the midst of a sick organization, culture or biosphere? Does it make sense to focus on the health of individuals while simultaneously ignoring our biological and cultural context?

The short answer is completely unsatisfactory. Yes, it is possible, for a time, to isolate individual bodies and promote individual adaptations. This is precisely what we see in the world of elite health clubs and athletics. Wealthy individuals channel a massive stream of energy and resources to themselves and so, in the short term, manage to build up islands of health. But this apparent health is not particularly meaningful, enduring or interesting. Given enough resources, just about anyone can do it.

In fact, health islands are not a good model for a sustainably healthy future. Yes, we can direct vast amounts of time, expertise and resources into building up the state of isolated bodies, teams or athletic programs, but what exactly have we accomplished? Aside from pumping up the appearance, vitality and status of the "islanders," all we've really done is stretch the social health gradient, increasing the distance between the health-rich and the health-poor. Ultimately, the process becomes self-defeating as the islanders, fit and healthy as they might be, find themselves isolated in a world of declining health.

WHO'S HOLISTIC?

Our understanding of human continuity gives new meaning to the practice of holistic health. In conventional circles, we typically label mind-body-spirit orientations as "holistic." But if we're only talking about *my* body, *my* mind and *my* spirit, what we're doing isn't even close to being holistic. In fact, when the mind-body-spirit orientation is focused on the individual, the best we can hope for is a temporary, unsustainable health island.

If we really want to be holistic, we have to include the rest of the biological and social world in our efforts. In this respect, the conventional prescription for health must be expanded to include diet, exercise and activism, intentional efforts towards preserving that which sustains us. In other words, watch what you eat, get off the couch and start being inconvenient. Eat real food, practice functional movement and stand up for environmental preservation, sustainable agriculture, peace and social justice. Take care of your internal organs, of course, but take care of your external organs too. It's all one body.

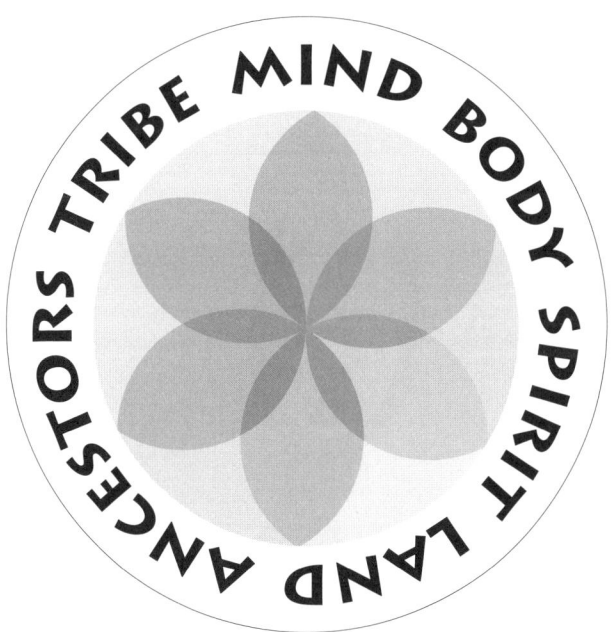

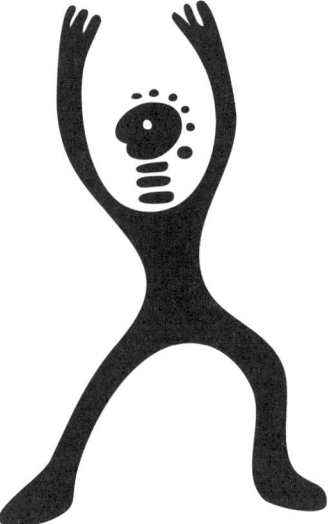

Change Your Body, Change the World

PRIMAL CONFUSION

> What is more important for us, at an elemental level, than the control, the owning and operation of our own physical selves?
>
> Olive Sacks
> *The Man Who Mistook His Wife for a Hat*

> There is only one core issue for all psychology: Where is the "me?" Where does the "me" begin? Where does the "me" stop?
>
> James Hillman
> *Ecopsychology*

> It is a terrible thing to see and have no vision.
>
> Helen Keller

My friends tell me that I'm just a hairy bag of water and I guess they must be right. Actually, I'm not really that hairy, but as for the water, that's true enough. All of us are aquatic organisms by nature, bubbles of moisture enclosed in an envelope of skin. When our ancestors crawled out of the ocean millions of years ago, they figured out a way to take the ocean with them. Metabolism just works better in a liquid medium. Thus, the bag.

Of course there's more to an organism than a hairy sack. Our bags need a musculoskeletal system to get around, feet for locomotion and hands for grasping. We need digestion to give us fuel and a nervous system to coordinate our activity and behavior, all so that the bag can get around in the world and send its genes into the future.

That's a start, but how will your bag know the nature of its world? How will it navigate or make decisions about gravity, terrain, obstacles, plants and animals? Will the bag just blunder about its world or will it make intelligent choices that allow it to survive in a dynamic and sometimes hostile environment?

SENSATION: WHAT'S IT GOOD FOR?

To meet this need, our bags come equipped with a set of incredibly sophisticated senses that provide an immense amount of information about the environment and the condition of the hairy bag itself. Multiple channels of data stream into our nervous systems, giving us the capability to direct our actions in ways that are appropriate to our surroundings.

Unfortunately, most of us fail to appreciate just how big a role sensation plays in our physical and psychological health. To get the whole story, we need to make a crucial distinction between somatic and special senses. These two types of senses have entirely different purposes and affect our experience in radically different ways.

The somatic senses are the oldest and most basic type. They tell us the intimate details about the state of our bodies: touch, thermoreception (hot and cold), nociception (pain), proprioception (position and movement in space) and balance (inner ear). Taken together, these somatic receptors give us a sense of our physical identity. In a very real sense, they tell us who we are.

In contrast, the special senses include vision, hearing, smell and taste. These senses are obviously important in managing our experience in the world, but as we shall see, their role is somewhat overrated.

A SPECIAL DEFICIT

To get an idea of the relative importance of the senses, we have only to think of people who are deprived of one type or the other. For example, consider the life of Helen Keller.

Most everyone knows the story: Born in 1880 with normal sensation, she was struck by scarlet fever or meningitis at age nineteen months. The illness did not last long, but it left her deaf and blind, a knockout blow to her special senses. Her somatic senses were left intact.

Keller's teacher arrived a few years later and began to teach her to communicate by spelling words into her hand. The breakthrough came when Keller realized that the motions that her teacher was making on the palm of her hand, while running cool water over her other hand, represented the idea of *water*.

Once she understood the nature of symbols, Keller began a passionate quest for knowledge and went on to become an extremely successful author, political activist and lecturer. She learned Braille and used it to read, not only in English but also French, German, Greek, and Latin. She wrote books and traveled the world, inspiring people wherever she went. She was the first deaf-blind person to earn a Bachelor of Arts degree. Most of us would be delighted to function at so high a level.

Keller's life teaches us many important lessons of course, but here we are particularly interested in her experience with sensation. For Keller, the loss of special senses was a tremendous challenge, but it was not insurmountable; she managed to flourish in spite of her deficit. Her identity, personality and sense of personal integration remained intact. Her life is proof that the special senses, while obviously desirable, are not absolutely essential for health and function.

"THE DISEMBODIED LADY"

In contrast, consider a story recounted by Oliver Sacks in *The Man Who Mistook His Wife for a Hat*. Sacks writes of a woman named Christian who lost her proprioception, her sense of body position and motion. Christian suffered a rare but debilitating case of "sensory neuritis," an inflammation of her sensory nerves. Almost overnight, she lost her awareness of her body and her sense of physical self. Not surprisingly, the effect was profoundly disturbing to her identity. Sacks described her predicament this way:

> She continues to feel, with the continuing loss of proprioception, that her body is dead, not-real, not-hers; she cannot appropriate it to herself. She can find no words for this state, and can only use analogies derived from other senses: 'I feel my body is blind and deaf to itself…it has no sense of itself—these are her own words.'

Ultimately, Christian's predicament proved to be far more difficult and tragic than Keller's. Although she was able to see and hear, she had no sense of physical identity. Her body had disappeared from her awareness.

After eight years of physical therapy, Christian showed no signs of neurological recovery and remained in a disembodied state. She learned to visually monitor her physical movements, but the process required highly disciplined, intentional concentration from moment to moment. She learned to walk and take public transport, but only with great effort and vigilance. At the time that Sack's book was published, it was unclear whether she ever regained a sense of personal identity or well-being.

THE DEMISE OF THE SOMATIC SENSES

Clinical curiosities are one thing; we might be inclined to write Christian's story off as an anomaly. But we can also see Christian's body-blind experience as an extreme example of an epidemic that is sweeping the modern world. That is, we have a huge population of individuals whose special senses are intact, but whose somatic senses are severely atrophied because of disuse.

The modern world robs us of somatic experience and sensation. Our sense of touch is diminished almost to the point of non-existence. Shoes and buildings insulate us from the earth and we lose an immense amount of sensory stimulation, starting at an early age. Modern homes and workplaces are constructed of smooth, monotonous materials. Where our hands once touched dirt, rocks, sticks and animal hides, they now touch texture-free countertops, desks, furniture and tools. To make matters even worse, social norms often discourage physical contact with other human bodies. For many of us, handshakes are the most intimate physical contact that we experience on any given day.

Proprioception and balance similarly fall into disuse and atrophy. Monotonous sidewalks, floors and stairways offer little stimulation to the body's position senses. Consequently, these sensory systems stop firing. We don't use the capability, so we lose it.

Our experience of hot and cold is also compromised. Most modern buildings are maintained at a constant 68 degrees. Synthetic clothing wicks moisture away from the skin and leaves us comfortable year round. Unless we're active in the outdoors, we may go weeks or months without feeling hot or cold.

Pain also diminishes. Our highly-engineered homes and workplaces are designed to eliminate scrapes, bumps, bruises, lacerations and other minor skin insults that are common in outdoor environments. To be sure, many people experience musculoskeletal pain, but these pains often come from other sources: sedentary postures, movement specializations and repetitive overuse.

PRIMAL CONFUSION

The atrophy of the somatic senses plays out in some disturbing patterns of human psychology, identity and behavior. For many in today's world, the body no longer feels itself clearly. Physical identity begins to weaken and drift. Without somatic sensation, we tend to forget who we really are. This becomes a state of "primal confusion."

The most obvious manifestations of this state are the ADD and ADHD that we see in so many of today's children, but it also shows up in a host of sub-clinical syndromes, in adults as well as children. Somatic sensory deprivation leads to anxiety, loss of concentration and poor performance. Without a sense of body, our minds and spirits begin to wander. We seek a sense of grounding anywhere we can, sometimes in substance abuse, excessive eating, chronic exercise, over-stimulation of the special senses or in some cases, cutting our own flesh.

Vigorous whole-body movement is a powerful antidote to this primal confusion because it floods the nervous system with primal sensation. The entire musculoskeletal system, in addition to getting us around in the world, also functions as a powerful sensory system. Every muscle, tendon and ligament is wired with mechanoreceptors that feed immense amounts of information back into the nervous system, telling us about the position of our bodies. The more we move, the more information we gather and the more integrated our bodymind begins to feel.

When we look at it from this perspective, we begin to realize that movement deprivation is also a form of sensory deprivation. Sedentary living doesn't just lead to muscular atrophy, it also leads to sensory atrophy. And in turn, this sensory atrophy leads to problems of cognition, attention, concentration and identity.

This is no trivial matter; sensory deprivation is widely recognized as a serious challenge to psychological well-being. In small doses, such as temporary immersion in a flotation tank, sensory deprivation may promote relaxation and creativity, but extended periods can produce extreme anxiety, hallucinations, depression and psychosis. In fact, sensory deprivation is sometimes used by the CIA to interrogate prisoners. The comparison is unavoidable: by living sedentary lives of sensory deprivation, we effectively torture ourselves.

SENSORY REBALANCING

So what is the solution to our epidemic of sensory amnesia and distortion? How shall we rediscover our bodies?

The short answer is to cut back on the visual stimulation and get back to some raw physical experience. Here's a prescription:

- More barefoot walking.
- More scrambling in the mountains.
- More exposure to dirt, trees and bushes.
- More massage.
- More sex.
- More rock climbing, rugby and martial art.
- More gardening, carpentry and woodworking.

And above all, more outdoor movement, especially multi-plane, multi-joint, exuberantly playful movement.

You just might rediscover your physical self.

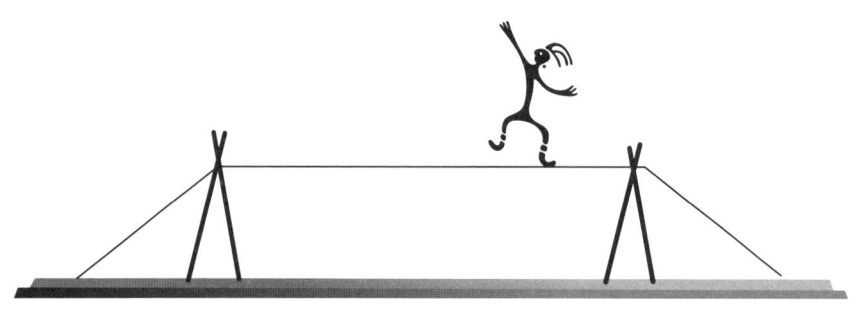

SEE THE LIGHT

> The precision of entrainment is vital if the organism is to be at peak performance.
>
> Russell Foster and Leon Kreitzman
> *Rhythms of Life: The Biological Clocks that Control the Daily Lives of Every Living Thing*

If you're like most health-curious people, you're looking to create a holistic experience for yourself, one that offers benefits to mind, body and spirit. Chances are you've spent a lot of time studying nutrition and movement and maybe you've included some stress education as well. That's a good start, but if you really want to make things comprehensive, you've got to add in another essential element: light.

Light is usually underrated as a factor in human health, but we are now coming to understand just how crucial it is in guiding our physiology, psychology and performance. Recent discoveries in chronobiology are revealing the power of light in health, disease and happiness. Light acts as a master regulator, tuning and synchronizing every process in the human body.

The story begins as it usually does, deep in human prehistory, on the semi-wooded grasslands of East Africa. Over the course of thousands of generations, our bodies were bathed in regular cycles of natural light and darkness. Humans are equatorial animals, evolved to live in an environment where daylight and darkness are roughly 12 hours each, all year round. Our entire hunting and gathering lifestyle was built around the position of the sun. Every action and movement was linked to light conditions (only a fool goes hunting at night or during the heat of mid-day). Ultimately, our health became inextricably linked to cycles of illumination.

But today we find ourselves in an alien circadian environment, a world in which our physiology is scrambled by chaotic patterns of non-natural light. This condition is now proving to be a far greater challenge to the human body than previously realized. In the years to come, trainers, therapists and body professionals of all sorts are going to be waking up to the importance of circadian health.

THE MASTER RHYTHM

When it comes to understanding the fundamentals of the human body, the key point to keep in mind is that all animal physiology is fundamentally rhythmic and that one master rhythm holds sway over every other—the circadian, day-night rhythm. All organisms on earth are driven by circadian cycles.

To make a long story short, the circadian nature of our bodies comes down to a simple bit of neuroanatomy. That is, the human brain comes equipped with a circadian pulse generator called the SCN (suprachiasmatic nucleus). This astounding bit of tissue consists of a mere 20,000 neurons that keep a circadian beat, roughly timed to 24 hours.

This is plenty astonishing in its own right, but even more fascinating is the fact that this endogenous pulse generator is only a blunt timing instrument that approximates the earth's circadian cycle. To manage physiology effectively, it needs to be fine-tuned (entrained) by actual environmental conditions, specifically by direct exposure to natural sunlight.

The crux of the problem is that our modern world provides weak, ineffective cues to day-night cycles. Unnatural light sources scramble our physiological rhythms and wreak all sorts of downstream havoc with our health and fitness. From the modern body's point of view, it is almost as if dawn and dusk are constantly shifting in random, arbitrary patterns.

It's no wonder our bodies are confused; we are literally cue-less. The problem is most pronounced in those of us who try to live on the wrong side of the clock: shift workers, airline pilots and college students, for example. But even for those who practice a roughly diurnal lifestyle, things can still go astray. We stay up late into the night and/or get up before dawn. We watch television and live in front of computers. Even when we're awake during the day, we expose ourselves to artificial lights that are simply too weak to entrain our biological clocks. Objects and surfaces under outdoor sunlight are illuminated at about 5000 to 100,000 lux, but indoor illumination is only 50 to 500 lux.

Clearly, the light coming off a computer screen is no substitute for the sun and it's no surprise that our rhythms tend to drift. Ultimately, the result is physiological mischief and deep physical confusion.

TIMING IS EVERYTHING

The implications of chronobiology for health and fitness practices are immense. For example, consider our encounters with food, dietary supplements or drugs. We now know that such substances have different effects when administered at different times of the day. For example, Foster and Kreitzman describe a study that tested cancer patients' responses to chemotherapy. The trial divided patients into two groups: each received the same drugs at the same dosages, but at different times of day. One group developed far fewer side effects: less hair loss, less nerve damage, less kidney damage, less bleeding and fewer transfusions. According to the lead researcher, "Every toxicity was markedly diminished several-fold simply depending on what time of day the drugs were given." (see "Circadian timing of cancer chemotherapy." *Science* 228, 73–75)

If we stop to think about it, this finding makes perfect sense. If physiology is constantly in flux, there are bound to be variations in response to substances that the body encounters. What's toxic in the morning might actually be therapeutic in the afternoon and vice-versa. A glass of wine at 6:00 pm may give you a warm, healthy glow, but at 11:00 pm it could disrupt your sleep.

As for substances, so too for physical movement. It's safe to assume that a hard sweaty workout will have dramatically different effects at different times of the day. And it's probably the case that, given enough knowledge, we will ultimately be able to customize the timing of our training sessions to achieve particular outcomes. If a person has diabetes, high blood pressure or depression, there is probably a best time of day for that person to train, dance or play.

Heraclitus was right of course: you can't step into the same river twice. The river of physiology is always changing and pulsing. As students of the body, we are taught that homeostasis is the body's prime directive, but this is only half the story. The body drives towards a stable equilibrium to be sure, but it also seeks synchronization with the oscillations of the environment and habitat. Thus, my physiology is varies throughout each day; I have a sunrise physiology, a mid-day physiology and an evening physiology. I am constantly rearranging my tissue in waves of anabolic and catabolic activity.

For the moment, we can build on a few key findings. For example, we know that tissue repair peaks between midnight and 4:00 am. ("Go to bed!") We know that concentration, logical reasoning and alertness are at their lowest between 4:00 and 6:00 am ("Take your time waking up.") We know that heart efficiency, muscle strength and flexibility are all highest between 4:00 and 8:00 pm. ("Try for your personal best in the late afternoon.") With experience, we will ultimately be able to tune our activity to match up with these circadian realities. And, in progressive, body-friendly workplaces and schools, managers will also begin to take circadian cycles into account.

GET OUT!

Chronobiology is a hot field that holds incredible promise for refining our approaches to the human body. Unfortunately, not enough people are taking it seriously. Aside from sporadic interest in jet-lag, shift work and seasonal affective disorder, very few professionals are integrating the discoveries of chronobiology into their practices. Very few physicians or pharmacists instruct patients on when to take medications for example, and scarcely any trainers are scheduling their sessions to match up with circadian realities. And in the world of big fitness, modern health clubs show blatant disregard for time of day. With constant levels of illumination in 24-hour facilities, every hour is the same as every other hour.

As exercisers, we find the principles of chronobiology to be both exhilarating and perplexing. We're excited by the promise of bringing our bodies into better harmony with circadian cycles and in the process, improving our physiological function, performance and maybe even our happiness. But the body is a moving target and this makes our job difficult. Not only do we have to provide high-quality movement experience and motivation to people, we have to do it at the right time of day.

Over the course of the next several decades, we will ultimately have the knowledge to craft training programs that are chronologically appropriate for every person. But in the meantime there are some simple steps that we can take to entrain our physiological rhythms. First and most important, do whatever you can to get out into the morning light. Think of outdoor light as an essential nutrient. If you can find a way to get outside, do it.

At least once a year, take an outdoor adventure that's highly circadian. For example, backpacking tends to be a truly in-your-face circadian experience. When the sun goes down, it gets cold and you snuggle into your bag. And as soon as it starts to get light, you're up again. Live this cycle for a few days and you'll be re-synchronized and ready to head back to the alien environment, refreshed and invigorated.

THE CASE AGAINST EXERCISE

> An hour of basketball feels like 15 minutes. An hour on a treadmill feels like a weekend in traffic school.
>
> David Walters

> The beginning of wisdom is the definition of terms.
>
> Socrates

So you've been on the couch for the last couple of decades and one day you wake up, look in the mirror and recoil in disgust. You're shocked at what you see and disturbed by what you feel. Disgusted with your lumpy, spongy form and its appalling lack of function, you resolve to turn things around, get back on track and whip yourself into shape. Your desperate mind searches for a remedy and quickly seizes upon a solution. That's right, you're going to exercise!

Swept up in a fever of enthusiasm, you launch yourself out the door. You buy some new workout clothes, fill your bag with supplements and sign up for a program at the local gym. You're ready to seize control of your fate and make a comeback.

But sadly, your mission will almost certainly fail, possibly within days, but definitely within months. If you're like most people, you're going to wind up back on the couch before you know it, nursing a beer and crafting a rationalization.

You might be tempted to blame your failure on a lack of resolve or a deficiency of willpower. But in fact, the real issue is that you called the thing by the wrong name. That's right, you used the word *exercise*. If you had thought things through a little more carefully, you might have realized that what you really needed was not exercise as such, but more physical *movement*.

To some, this may sound like a case of semantic hair-splitting, but there's actually a vital difference here, one that's lost on most Americans as well as a great many coaches, trainers and PE teachers. Understanding this distinction will take us a long way toward regaining our lost physicality and might even improve our relationship with the world at large.

EXERCISE IS ABNORMAL

The problem with exercise becomes apparent as soon as we begin to describe it. That is, exercise consists of doing abstracted movements in a stereotyped, repetitive pattern. In essence, exercise is a specialization extracted from a larger whole, an activity taken out of its natural context. Just as white flour is an extract derived from a more complex natural grain (losing most of its nutritional value in the process), exercise is a behavior that is stripped down and removed from its original setting. In effect, exercise is *white movement*.

When we stand back to take the long view of human history, we begin to see that exercise constitutes only a tiny fraction of the human movement repertoire. Our physical experience actually includes a vast range of kinetic behavior: locomotion and exploration, play, hunting, gathering, scavenging, climbing, sex, dance, labor, gesturing and expression. Exercise is only a very recent and minor subset of all possible human movements.

Exercise also stands out as a glaring exception in the natural world. Across the entire range of non-human animals, we see no behavior that resembles exercise, especially in the wild. Yes, rodents will run on wheels in their cages, but this is mostly a matter of incarceration and frustration; put a running wheel into a natural, grassy field and rodents will *not* be lining up to run on it. In wild settings, animals will play, hunt, graze, explore, fight and mate, but they never exercise. Even chimps and bonobos, our closest primate relatives, don't display anything that looks like our version of exercise. They get plenty of action playing, exploring and chasing one another around the forest.

The main problem with exercise is that it's all about sets, reps and mileage: just keep grinding it out until the clock runs out or your trainer tells you to stop. This, of course, is a recipe for physical monotony. And physical monotony, like any kind of repetitive behavior, tends to be hard on both the mind and tissue. Keep stressing a joint, tendon or ligament in an identical pattern and you'll promote inflammation and a lasting relationship with your physical therapist. Even worse, this sensory-motor monotony soon leads to a deeper, more disturbing psychospiritual monotony. Boredom sets in and the spirit becomes depressed. Resignation and apathy soon follow.

At the same time, exercise also fails because stereotyped reps tend to drive out play. This is why it's so hard to get kids to exercise. Their bodies are simply too smart to allow it. Treadmills are boredom machines; no healthy child will spend more than a few minutes on one.

The contrast is clear: exercise is about repetition of known patterns while play is about exploration and discovery. Exercise is about enduring unpleasant sensation; play is about finding delight in diverse movement forms. Exercise is about repeating the known; play is about extending into the unknown. Exercise requires external motivation to maintain participation; play is inherently rewarding and self-reinforcing.

Because of its repetitive, predictable and unpleasant nature, exercise ultimately takes on an adversarial tone and becomes a pitched battle of us against the experience. Faced with the prospect of mind-body monotony, we start looking for motivation and incentives. Thus, the proliferation of boot camps, TVs, carrots and sticks that we now bring to the modern gym. We've even taken to programming artificial voices of encouragement into treadmills, stairclimbers and other exercise machines. And so, exercise ultimately makes a perfectly logical companion to that other famously adversarial health experience: dieting.

A NON-SOLUTION

Exercise is commonly promoted as a cure for everything that ails our bodies and our spirits: obesity, diabetes, heart disease, depression and all the rest. "Just do more exercise" is the common prescription offered by both professionals and well-meaning friends.

But if exercise were actually the solution to our public health crisis, wouldn't we be seeing better results? After all, experts and celebrities have been promoting exercise for decades and the state of the human body continues to deteriorate. In fact, if we look at the trajectories of human lifestyle disease and exercise promotion, we would see that they track pretty closely with one another. Looking strictly at correlation, we might even come to the conclusion that exercise promotion *causes* atrophy, obesity, depression and poor health.

Exercise advocates are quick to point to success stories. We hear about pounds lost, blood sugar normalized, heart disease prevented and bodies transformed. We hear about people who fought mightily against physical apathy and dragged themselves to the gym for weeks, months and years. And yes, they showed impressive resolve and they got results.

What we rarely hear about are the multitudes of people who tried exercise, found it to be a dreadful bore and dropped out. In fact, the entire health club business model is built upon the assumption that a substantial proportion of members will stop attending shortly after signing the contract. In other words, failure is assumed.

In short, exercise has been a spectacular public health failure and an immense waste of human potential. The biggest consequence of exercise promotion is that we have managed to make millions of people feel guilty about their failure to do something that is inherently unpleasant.

START A MOVEMENT MOVEMENT

So exercise fails. Do we have a better idea?

Yes, in fact we do: authentic, joyful, functional movement.

For those who have never seen or experienced it, authentic movement looks and feels nothing like exercise. Here's the difference:

- Exercise tends to be single-plane; functional movement is multi-joint and multi-plane.
- Exercise is monotonous; movement is engaging.
- Exercise is specialized; movement is diverse.
- Exercise is scripted; movement is spontaneous and opportunistic.
- Exercise feels mechanized and forced; movement feels expressive and creative.
- Exercise is a means towards an end; movement is an end in itself.

Movement is better because it offers more options for physical creativity and expression. There's more possibility and more room for the imagination. It's more inviting and less adversarial.

OFF THE COUCH

So maybe it's time to head out for a walk and re-think your entire mission statement for the coming year. Your best bet is to give up on exercise right now; you'd be doing that soon enough anyway. Instead, resolve to get more movement into your life, by any means possible.

Of course, this emphasis on movement over exercise doesn't get us off the hook: vigorous physical engagement is still essential if we want to improve or maintain our health. If we want to reap the health and performance rewards, sweat and exertion are still necessary We still need to challenge our tissue and push our physical comfort zones.

So start by diversifying your efforts. Be a movement opportunist; look for movement at home, in the workplace, in parks, airports and in the parking lot. But most importantly, look for dance. Dance with terrain, with gravity and with other human bodies. Dance with dumbbells, kettlebells and sticks. Dance with imaginary opponents and shadows on the ground. Dance with water, with bushes and with trees. Dance with boulders, rocks and alpine ridges. Dance with stairs and sidewalks.

And remember, if it feels monotonous and boring, it probably *is* monotonous and boring. If this is the case, stop doing it! There are countless variations, combinations and permutations of movements that are engaging and exhilarating. So mess around, play with the possibilities until you find a combination of movement, speed, resistance and frequency that works for you.

You just might find a physical lifestyle that's truly sustainable.

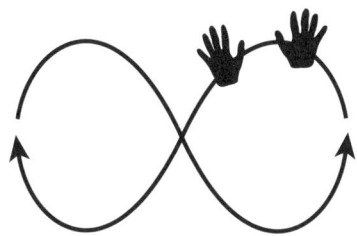

FIGURE EIGHTS:
ALL SIZES, STANCES AND SPEEDS

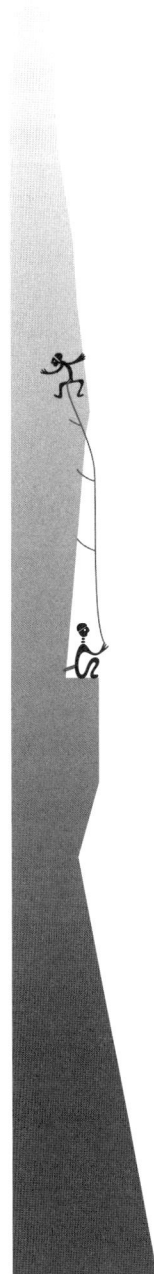

Change Your Body, Change the World

PUMPED TO PERFECTION

Nature is ever at work building and pulling down, creating and destroying, keeping everything whirling and flowing, allowing no rest but in rhythmical motion, chasing everything in endless song out of one beautiful form into another.

John Muir

It would be reasonable to say that everything that happens in our bodies is rhythmic until proven otherwise.

Josephine Arendt, neurobiologist

If you've ever traveled the rock climbing circuit of North America, you've probably been struck by the multitude of creative and fanciful route names at every cliff and crag. Every crack, face and corner has a name bestowed upon it by the first ascent party. These unique names give a sense of story, history and color to the climbing culture.

There are thousands of names in the guidebooks, but one stands out as iconic for our entire physical enterprise: *In Search of the Perfect Pump*. It's a fun name for a route because it captures the quest for peak physical experience. It's fascinating to hear climbers—connoisseurs of physical experience—talk about their pursuit:

> "Yeah dude, that pitch was way rad and it felt really killer, but if that layback was just a little bit longer, I could have gotten even more pumped."

> "I know, man, like it was really sick and pumpy at the crux, but then it got way casual with those big jugs over the roof."

"Yeah, it was kinda sketchy through that thin section and then it got rattly and there was nothing for the feet, but it just wasn't long enough to make it a mega-classic. The crux was too short and the holds were too big."

And on it goes for hours, around the campfire and in countless conversations on drives to and from the climbing area. These athletes are on a mission, always on the lookout for the ideal physical experience.

But what of it? Are these climbers simply physical zealots on a strange and fanatical mission? Why would people go half way around the world looking for the ideal climbing route that will pump their bodies to the ultimate level? What is it about "the perfect pump" that drives otherwise rational people to give up their jobs, their mates and sometimes their futures, all to go in search of an ideal physical experience? Is this just a quirky behavior of a minor subculture or are these people really on to something?

I believe these climbers are actually on a quest of profound importance, not just with regard to their own lives and health, but to the entire predicament of the modern human body. If more people went out looking for the ideal physical experience, our bodies would be a lot better off. Not only would we have radically reduced rates of cardiovascular disease, diabetes, obesity and depression, we'd see a big payoff in exuberance and happiness. We need this.

HOW DOES IT FEEL?

To find out what's so great about the perfect pump, let's have a closer look at the nature of the experience. To start, we might say that the perfect pump is characterized by high levels of metabolic efficiency and physiological integration: all systems of the body are operating at peak output and are tightly integrated. Muscular, respiratory, digestive, sensory and neuroendocrine performance is optimal.

Of course, this description is boring and fails to capture the true nature of the experience. For this, we need to listen to the connoisseurs, the romantics who thrive on the experience. When these athletes describe the perfect pump, they won't tell us about metabolic efficiency or metrics. Rather, they'll tell us how incredibly wonderful it feels. It's an integrated experience of mind, body, spirit and the creative imagination. It's massively physical to be sure, but also metaphysical.

Far more than a case of endorphin intoxication, the perfect pump is profoundly multi-dimensional. At is finest, it is magical, even transcendent. The body is pulsing with fatigue and exhilaration, heat and power. Vessels are dilated, fluids are flowing, membranes are vibrating, synapses are firing at high intensity. The body is surging beyond its normal capability and delights in the discovery of intense physicality. The spirit is swept up in the passion of the moment. The experience is raw, primal and in its own way, erotic. It's an ecstatic merger with life. It's unforgettable and highly addictive.

OUR PUMPY WORLD

This description draws us in and inspires us to try it for ourselves, but the appeal goes even deeper. The significance of the perfect pump multiplies as soon as we broaden our view of biology and physiology. Suddenly, we begin to see pumps everywhere: all living things are pulsing and pumping, vibrating and oscillating, continuously moving substances back and forth.

When we get right down to it, we begin to see that all organisms are pumps. In essence, pumping is what plants and animals do. We pump solids, liquids and gasses continuously throughout every second of our lives. We begin pumping at conception and don't stop pumping until the moment that we die. In fact, it would not be an exaggeration to say that life itself is a system of interconnected pumps.

Pumps are active at every level of biology. Cellular membranes pump substances back and forth, bringing nutrients in and pushing wastes out. Digestive pumps operate beneath consciousness, squeezing organs and tubes as they move solids and liquids. Vascular tissue pumps blood throughout the body while muscular diaphragms pump gasses in and out. At the same time, the oceans, atmosphere and major biomes are all pumping on a massive scale. Forests, grasslands and marshes pump heat, moisture and gasses. Even the geologic foundation of the earth, the tectonic plates, are slowly surging and drifting, pulsing to the beat of magma that surges between them. The entire biosphere, even the universe itself perhaps, is pulsing.

BEYOND HOMEOSTASIS

As it turns out, pumping is right at the core of metabolism, both within and beyond the body. If you think back to your early classroom studies of the body, you'll probably remember being told that homeostasis was the prime directive of physiology and in turn, health itself. The "wisdom of the body" is that it strives to keep a constant *internal milleu,* a stable environment inside the cell and inside the body. A constant balancing act of countervailing forces, the body manages to keep itself poised between *hyper* and *hypo.*

This boilerplate explanation is a start, but it neglects the larger story. That is, this apparent stability of physiology is actually the product of motion. The corrective powers that exist within the organism can only be brought to bear when solids, liquids and gasses are flowing. Thus, pumping becomes essential to homeostasis and stability. Regular oscillations of limbs, tissues, membranes and fluids are what make homeostasis possible. Without pumping action, physiology breaks down and health goes with it.

PUMP FOR HEALTH

At this point, we can make some solid assumptions about the nature of the thing that we call "health." That is, the stronger the pump and its component sub-pumps, the healthier the organism. The weaker the pumps, the more health is at risk. In fact, we could even condense all our health advice to a single formula for better living: promote the pump.

The good news is that physiological pumps become increasingly effective when challenged with vigorous use. This is the SAID principle: Specific Adaptation to Imposed Demands. We impose a demand on the organism by asking it to increase its pumping activity; we run uphill or climb big rocks and drive the pump to exhaustion. Repeat this process over the course of a few weeks and the pumping mechanism becomes more efficient. The organism learns how to move stuff around more efficiently, especially fluids. Pump capability increases and so does health. It's a tried and true formula for success.

In fact, knowing the value of pumping in health, we might even begin to revisit some of our long-held assumptions about exercise. That is, we're starting to understand that the whole concept of "exercise" is too vague. Rather than simply moving our bodies with no particular goal in mind, we'd all be better off if we went in search of a powerful, fluid-moving experience.

NESTED PUMPS: HARMONIZING AND SYNCHRONIZING

Most health advocates understand the importance of pumpy movement and its role in maintaining vitality, but the story is actually more intricate and fascinating than it might first appear.

Despite superficial appearances, the human body is not a stand-alone pump. Rather, it functions within an ecosystem that is itself an immensely powerful collection of interconnected pumps. We are a nested pump within a vast set of interconnected pumping systems. There's the circadian pump, the seasonal pump, the annual pump. Each of these pumpy oscillations has powerful effects on the functioning of the entire organism.

So, it's not enough to train your body to be a strong and effective stand-alone pump. Our individual pumping needs to be harmonized and synchronized with the other pumps in our world. Timing, beat and rhythm are crucial.

Unfortunately, the modern world compromises our pumps in several ways. First and most obviously, it weakens our individual pumping capabilities through sedentary behavior. Pumps, like all body tissues and functions, atrophy with neglect. In effect, sedentary bodies forget how to move fluid. Metabolism slows. Turnover of nutrients and waste products becomes weaker and tissues begin to suffer.

Even worse, modern living drives us into unsynchronized patterns of activity, completely at odds with natural oscillations. We pump our bodies arbitrarily or at the service of artificial schedules that have nothing to do with environmental conditions. We pump our bodies at the wrong times of day, in the wrong seasons and at the wrong intensities. Consequently, our pumping capability, even if individually strong, falls out of rhythm with larger pumps.

ELEMENTS OF THE PERFECT PUMP

Given what we know about the vital importance of the pump, it's time to talk about the elements of the perfect body-pumping experience. Obviously, there will be huge individual variation here; one person's perfect pump will be another person's day at the beach and yet another person's worst nightmare. Some will lean towards endurance, others towards strength, still others towards skill. Since we all come with our own unique genetics and physical history, it makes sense that we would seek out our own customized experiences. That said, there is a consensus as to what characterizes a perfect pump. Most connoisseurs agree that the experience includes these core elements:

EXERTION

Without question, there must be a serious physical effort involved; the entire organism must be challenged. This may be through exposure to natural forces—as in climbing—or through simple, honest physical commitment to any physical experience. In any case, it's about pushing the outer limits of one's comfort zone. Doubt is an essential part of the process. If you know you can do it, it's less likely to be a perfect pump.

HEAVY BREATHING

Second, the perfect pump has to involve the cardiovascular system in a big way. Heavy breathing, sweat and oxygen debt are essential. If your diaphragm and intercostal muscles aren't heaving, it's not a perfect pump. This means big body movements and major participation by big muscle groups. Think uphill running.

By the same token, a single-repetition squat or bench press cannot qualify, no matter how much weight you put on the bar. Similarly, golf can never be a perfect pump. If there's no load on the cardiovascular system, there's no pumping going on.

POWER-ENDURANCE

Of the common athletic events, middle distance is most likely to produce a perfect pump. A 100 meter sprint is too short, a marathon is too long. But a 440 or 880 is awesomely pumpy. When you cross the finish line, your chest will be heaving and your entire body will know itself in a new way.

Similarly, short reps with big weights or long reps with light weights fail to produce a perfect pump. The mid-range combination of reps and weight, when pushed to the end range of an individual's capability, moves a lot of fluid and qualifies as the ideal pump. Medicine balls are ideal for this purpose.

HIPS

Another key element in the perfect pump is involvement of the hips. The hip joints are the largest joints in the body and have enormous pumping capacity. When quads and butt participate in vigorous, high-amplitude oscillations, fluid flow between the legs and trunk increases dramatically. Big, deep movements have the most potential. The trick is to bend your knees and get down in your stance. Squats and squat-like variations are ideal.

MULTI-SENSORY

Ideally, the perfect pump will involve the entire sensorium. It will be heavily visual, auditory and even olfactory, but most importantly, it will be highly tactile. That is, the skin must get into the act. Hands, feet, arms and legs are all touching the world in some way, receiving information and generating physical knowledge.

To experience this sensory element, it is essential to remove anything that would stand in its way. This means abandoning the iPod and other acoustic distractions; this is not a time for entertainment.

Similarly, if you can possibly go barefoot, do it. Expose your body to the experience in every way possible. This is the time for a true physical encounter and embrace, not for insulation.

OUTDOORS

Finally, the perfect pump should take place outdoors in natural conditions. Only in nature can we synchronize our individual pumping bodies with the larger biological pumps of which we are a part. Natural light, terrain and textures are essential to the complete experience. Indoor cycling, no matter how sweaty, can never be a perfect pump. Indoor yoga, martial art, or weight lifting are all worth doing, but they can never be truly complete. If you want your pump to work in harmony with the rest of the living world, you need to put your body in contact with powerful environmental forces.

GET THE "WHY" RIGHT

The basic elements of the perfect pump are simple. Just choose an activity that's got a big cardio demand, a big muscular demand and do it outdoors in a natural setting. If you customize it to your personal preferences and push it hard, you'll approach a perfect pump.

The more subtle skill lies in getting the motivation right. This is critical. Consensus, at least in the worlds of rockclimbing and surfing, is that the quest should be pursued for its own sake, not as a means to some achievement. The perfect pump should be an experience unto itself. We are seeking a transcendent physical moment-in-time, completely independent of future goals. It's the quality that matters most and that quality can only happen in the present.

Yes, there will be health benefits. And yes, your athletic performance will almost certainly improve, especially if your pumpy training aligns with your chosen sport. But these future benefits can be distractions that derail us from our original objective. Seek out the perfect pump, not because of what it will do for you in some abstract future, but because of what it will do for you today. Keep the focus on the aesthetics of the experience, not the payoff. A perfect pump is a beautiful thing in itself.

THE POTENTIAL

So, it turns out that the search for the perfect pump is not just a trivial quirk of a minor sporting sub-culture. Rather, it is a fundamental part of physical discovery and deserves to be taken seriously by all people, no matter what their physical capabilities. The beauty is that there's something for everyone here—an ideal pump exists for everyone, regardless of their physical state or capability.

Finding it will be the first challenge, of course. A coach or a trainer might give you some ideas, but ultimately it's up to your imagination. To find your perfect pump, start with the essential elements, then tweak to suit. Work around nagging injuries as necessary. If you knee hurts, look for the perfect core and upper-body pump. If you shoulder is lame, you can still run uphill. If in doubt, take a medicine ball outdoors and look for a hill; you should be able to come up with something.

In any case, the details are trivial. What's important is process. Seek out middle-distance, middle-load activities and push them hard. Get your whole body engaged and go after the activity with focused commitment. Drive it as hard as you can for a little bit longer than you think you can, then celebrate the sensation you've created. Relish the sweat, the surging breath, the flood of neurotransmitters. Celebrate the pulsing in your muscles, in your heart and in your spirit. It's a moment worth savoring.

THE ART OF THE ARC

In life, as in art, the beautiful moves in curves.

> Edward G. Bulwer-Lytton

Magic lives in curves, not angles.

> Mason Cooley

If you're curious about how the human body moves or how it might move better, you might be tempted to turn to one of those weighty anatomy or physiology textbooks. These impressive volumes give us all the information we could ever want about biomechanics and kinesiology, but unfortunately, the actual experience of graceful, powerful movement never really comes across. No matter how detailed and authoritative the content, such reference books fail to deliver what we're after; we can be sure that nobody has ever learned how to dance by reading a textbook on biomechanics.

Fortunately, we have some good alternatives in the world around us. Movement teachers begin by modeling with their own bodies of course, but they also refer to familiar objects with body-like characteristics: golf clubs, whips, bungee cords and other objects with a resilient, rebounding quality. For my part, I've chosen the fly rod, a structure that mimics the movement of the body particularly well. As an occasional angler, I've spent some pleasant days wielding this instrument and have had plenty of time to reflect on the way it mimics the qualities of the human arm.

Like a human limb, the fly rod is a resilient, elastic structure with a strong tendency to return to its neutral form. The rod has a gradient of flexibility and elasticity along its length: it's stiff at the base and flexible at the tip. This is similar to what we see in the human torso and extremities; the biggest muscles attach to a powerful base (the hips, pelvis and lumbar spine) and become progressively more flexible and delicate towards the hands and feet.

Of course, the fly rod is not a perfect match for all varieties of human movement. The body is capable of a vast number of movements with wildly different qualities: some short and explosive, others long and luxurious. The fly rod is useful because it represents one of the most classic examples of athletic power, grace and flow. It's a particularly close match to pitching or throwing, but the same principles apply to all human and animal movements.

THE BIOMECHANICS OF FLY FISHING

The most intriguing similarities between the fly rod and human movement come in the casting cycle. In the back-cast, the weight and momentum of the fishing line pull the elastic fibers of the rod into a stretch, which then rebound to pull the line forward in harmony with the contraction in the caster's arm.

In the language of biomechanics, the fly rod goes through two distinct phases of motion: a loading phase in which the elastic fibers come under stretch, followed by an active power phase in which the stored energy is released into movement. This is the same dynamic that takes place when a human limb moves through an athletic range of motion. Movement is decelerated, then accelerated. Force is reduced, then produced. In terms of their kinetic qualities, the fibers of the fly rod and the tissues of the human limb are doing almost precisely the same thing.

Of course, the fly rod is a passive structure; the microscopic fibers rebound like miniature bungee cords that return to their resting state. But imagine what would happen if, by some miracle of biotechnology, we were able to implant living contractile tissue into the fibers of the fly rod. This would have two effects. First, it would make the structure far more powerful; fishermen would love it because you could cast much farther. Second, it would give the angler much more opportunity for control. No longer would you have to go through a set range of motion to take all the slack out of the elastic fibers. Instead, you could store energy in the contractile fibers with whatever amount of back-cast you wanted.

At this point you'd have a really neat fly rod and you'd probably win some casting awards and catch some really big fish. But if you wanted the ultimate system, you'd want to incorporate a communication system—a nervous system—to help you manage and control the behavior of the contractile fibers. You'd want sensory fibers to monitor the position and movement of the contractile elements and you'd want motor fibers to provide just the right amount of stimulus to power the casting action. What's more, you'd want all of these sensory and motor fibers to interconnect in such a way as to integrate and orchestrate the total movement of the entire system. This, of course, is precisely what we see in the human body: elastic, contractile elements coordinated by a hyper-fast communication processing system.

STRETCHING AND STRENGTHENING

Once we understand the fly rod metaphor and the way that it resembles a human limb, we're in a better position to understand our own movement and make some intelligent choices about physical training. In particular, we're better able to understand things like stretching and strengthening.

For example, we begin to understand that the thing we call "strength" is not a single quality. Rather, it is a composite skill that includes sensation, movement management and neural drive. Every good lift is an orchestration of movement, a coordination of active and passive elements in the body. Every act of strength includes the movement that comes immediately before the lift itself. There's a pre-motion in which the limb is stretched and loaded, a transition phase in which elastic and contractile fibers change direction and a power phase in which motor neurons drive the movement. Mastery of this complete movement cycle is what defines strength.

When we study the kinetic chain as an orchestrated arc, it soon becomes obvious that isolated, bodybuilder-style training makes almost no sense for developing functional strength. Isolation training targets individual segments of the chain, but it does little for the chain as a whole. It does nothing to promote athletic communication or orchestration. In fact, it can actually wreck the functionality of the chain. If one segment becomes dominant over the others, the totality of the arc becomes distorted.

Just as the arc helps us to understand strength, it also helps us to understand the role of stretching. Once again, we start to think of the totality of the system and the integrated movement of the arc. It soon becomes obvious that there's an optimal range of motion for every joint. If a joint is too tight, it will force greater stress and hyper-mobility into the joints above and below it. If the joint is too loose, it will suffer repetitive stress and trauma.

Of course, the mobility of these joints depends on more than just passive tissue of the joints themselves; it is very much a function of neurological communication between sensory and motor neurons. The functional range of our joints is mediated by the "stretch reflex," a high-speed neural conversation that constantly adjusts position and motion.

This reflex has two functions. First, it's a protective mechanism that prevents over-stretch injuries to contractile tissues and inert tissues of joints (i.e. ligaments and joint capsules). In the fly rod, it would help to prevent overextending the back-cast, which would save wear and tear on the elastic fibers of the rod. Since the contractile fibers are stimulated when the reach maximum stretch, this would help to protect the integrity of the entire structure.

Second, the stretch reflex is a performance-enhancing mechanism that helps to coordinate and amplify the concentric contraction—the forward cast. For the fly rod, the reflex becomes active as the back-cast nears full range of motion. This makes for a more powerful and integrated forward motion.

So, the stretch reflex is a good friend; it keeps our bodies happy and helps us perform at a high level. We want it to fire powerfully and at the precise moment when it's needed. And we want it to work in harmony with the rest of the kinetic arc. Indiscriminate stretching, especially long-duration static holds, will not give us the result that we're looking for. If the stretch is consistently isolated to a particular segment, it can be counter-productive, producing hyper-mobility and distortion in the arc of movement. We are far better off to seek integrated, functional stretches that challenge the entire chain as a single system.

KINKS, FLAT SPOTS AND SENSORY-MOTOR AMNESIA

Not only does the arc of the fly rod help us to understand physical movement and training, it also helps us understand what happens in pain and injury. When things are working well, we see a smooth gradient of flexibility all along the movement arc: strong and stable at the base and progressively more mobile towards the tip. As long as it retains this gradient, it will continue to function at a high level.

But with injury, the kinetic chain begins to experience pain, stiffness or distorted mobility, especially at the joints. In effect, the chain develops kinks or flat spots. Even if you don't feel pain, you feel that something is awkward in your movements. At the very least, your skill is compromised. At worst, you start to have trouble executing basic tasks.

So what are these "kinks" in the arc of human movement? The most powerful explanation comes from an understanding of the sensory-motor nervous system. In an ideal state, every part of the kinetic chain is sending clear, loud sensory information to the spinal cord where data can be processed and returned in the form of motor commands. Every segment is awake, alive and communicating. This allows for constant dynamic adjustment across the entire chain.

But now suppose that one part of the chain goes quiet. Injury, fatigue, excess repetition or disuse may cause a segment to stop signaling. Or, the body's arcs might be disrupted by subtle psychosocial forces that act on posture and movement: the way we stand, sit or walk is often influenced by our experience in community. Whatever the original cause, some element drops out of the conversation, no longer sending clear content to the spinal cord and brain.

Without this sensory information, the motor system becomes confused. It is forced to take a guess and compensate for the lack of information. It begins to send motor commands to the wrong part of the chain or in the wrong intensity. The main actor (you) will still try to execute the movement you desire, but the chain just isn't working right, all because of a quiet, sleepy or inactive sensory segment in the chain. And now your movement arc develops kinks, flat spots, pain and dysfunction.

Thomas Hanna, the creator of Somatic Education, described these distortions in the movement arc as "sensory-motor amnesia." The phrase is a good one because it implies that some part of the movement arc has "forgotten" how to send the appropriate signals. Kinks, flat spots, pain and weakness are, first and foremost, a communication problem. In effect, parts of the system have "gone dark" and dropped out of the neurological conversation.

In popular conversation, we think about our bodies and the pain we experience in terms of simple injury. We take the anti-inflammatory medications and hope for relief. We ice, rest and complain, but often to no avail. But contrary to our experience, the pain itself may not be the problem. The pain is just a symptom of a dysfunctional system, a kinetic chain with a broken conversational pattern. Instead of working as an intelligent, integrated, orchestrated system, parts of the chain have become sleepy, slow or stupid.

This study of neural communication leads us to some fresh ideas about ideal function and performance. We might say that "a chain is only as strong as its weakest link" and let it go at that. But now, we might refine our idea to say "the arc is only as smooth as its slowest link. Or even better, "the arc is only as graceful as its poorest communicator."

REMEDIES

So what are we to do with the sleepy segments in our bodies that lead to sensory-motor confusion? How do we smooth out those kinks in the arc? How do we wake up elements that have lost their voice?

The primary goal is to bring attention and awareness to the dark, quiet spots in the arc of movement. A good place to begin is by slowing down. Reawaken the arc by paying close attention to micro-movements and subtleties. Can you feel every single element of the chain as it goes through movement? If not, slow down and try it again. This process takes time. It also helps to have a coach, a movement educator who's experienced in facilitating movement awareness.

Somatic educators advocate an intriguing approach to sensory-motor awareness called *pandiculation*. In sort, this is a yawn or yawn-like stretching movement. Yawns, of course, are short-duration stretches that effectively wake up the body; yawn-like movements effectively reset neuromuscular elements to their ideal length. This approach strikes us as profoundly natural: non-human animals never hold long-duration stretches in the wild, but they do *pandiculate* frequently throughout the day. To practice this art, look for yawn-like movements that act across long kinetic chains and pay close attention to the subtleties of how they feel.

Another approach is simply to try new movements. Novelty is inherently stimulating and might, if you're lucky, wake up some sleepy neural elements. This argues for a diversity of training, including play. Don't specialize too narrowly; get away from professionalized routines that simply dig sensory and motor ruts deeper and deeper. Instead, play around the fringes of your motor patterns. Do what you do, but do it with a different emphasis; change the speed, the quality, the range or the intent.

In the end, it's all about education, that is, bodymind self-education. It's a process that each of us must ultimately take responsibility for. Movement teachers can create the right environment, they can facilitate, they can offer suggestions and inspiration, but they cannot do the real work. This challenge will always fall to us.

GETTING THE KINKS OUT

The fly rod makes an interesting model for biomechanical function. It helps us understand how our bodies work and suggests effective methods for training and rehabilitation. But things get even more interesting if we use the movement arc as a metaphor for systems outside our bodies. What about kinks and dead spots in the rest of our lives? In our relationships, our families and our workplaces and our culture?

Surely there must be lessons as well. After all, these exterior relationships are organic, dynamic structures too. Maybe we can use what we know about the body's movement arc to inform our behavior at other levels.

It's impossible to prescribe specific solutions of course; every relationship, kink and dead spot in a system's arc is unique. Every flaw in communication, whether neurological, interpersonal, institutional or cultural, has its particular origins and history.

Nevertheless, we would do well to try the same principles at any level: Look for integration and orchestration of the entire arc of the relationship: take a systemic and holistic approach. Share the load across all the elements of the chain. Look for optimal range of motion in every segment; neither too stiff or too flexible. Emphasize communication and rapport between "sensory" and "motor" systems. Refine the flow of information within the system. Slow down to smarten up: find the sleepy segments and get them talking. Find the overactive, hyper-reactive segments and calm them down. Play with diversity of movement; try new patterns.

And if all else fails, get yourself a good fly rod and head out to a quiet lake or stream. You may not catch a single fish, but you can study the grace and beauty of the cast. The dynamism of the arc will refresh your understanding of naturally integrated movement and perhaps spark some new ideas. Marvel at the way the elements combine into powerfully coordinated movement. Integrate that lesson into your body and see what it does for the other arcs in your life.

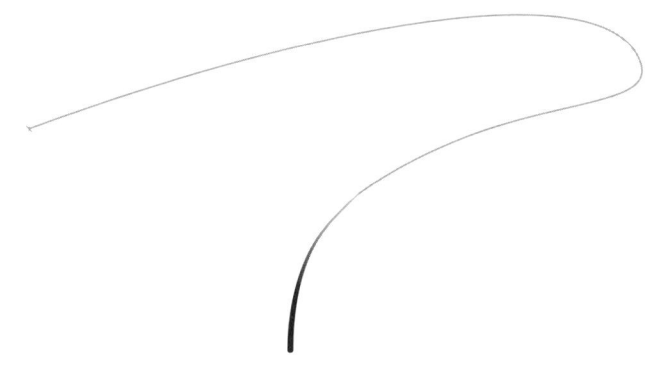

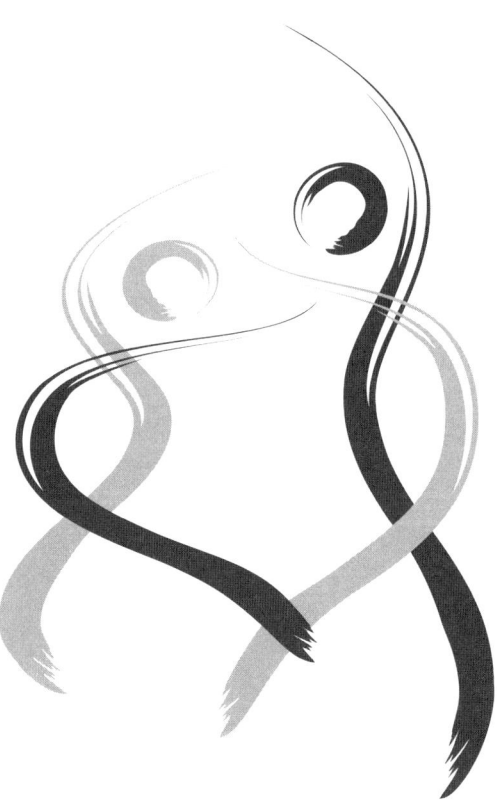

Change Your Body, Change the World

ROMANCING THE BODY

> We should take care not to make the intellect our god; it has, of course, powerful muscles, but no personality.
>
> Albert Einstein

> Pure logic is the ruin of the spirit.
>
> Antoine de Saint-Exupéry

So, you want to argue about physical training, health and the ways of the body? Well of course you do. Everyone has an opinion these days, and a lot of those opinions are strident, passionate and well-reasoned.

At first glance, our ideas seem to be all over the map, but on closer examination it turns out that there are really two distinct schools of thought on the life and conditioning of the body; one is classical, the other romantic.

To understand this distinction, let's take a trip back to some classic hippie literature of the 1960's: Robert Pirsig's *Zen and the Art of Motorcycle Maintenance*. Pirsig was a writer-philosopher and he probably wasn't in very good shape, but he did give us an incredibly useful distinction about our habits of thought, a distinction that we can apply directly to the predicament of the modern human body.

For Pirsig, the classic mode of thought is rational, linear, organized and sequential. We recognize the classic perspective when we hear people talk about systems, hierarchies, sequences, units, precision and quantity. Typically, we think of engineers, accountants and administrators. We also think of exercise scientists, physical therapists and biomechanical specialists. In contrast, we recognize the romantic perspective when we focus on experience, aesthetics, passion, wildness, sensation and quality. We think of artists, musicians, dancers, poets and lovers.

For the health and fitness enthusiast, it's easy to see these qualities in the ways that people approach exercise and conditioning. On one hand we have the romantic artist who's primarily interested in the quality of the movement experience. He speaks the language of passion, feeling, expression and inspiration. When he steps into the studio or the outdoors, he's looking to create an experience with meaning. For him, vigorous physical movement is considered an end in itself. (It's "auto-telic.") If it feels good, it is good.

On the other hand we have classically-oriented athletes who focus their attention on data, quantification and measurable results. When the classical exerciser steps into the gym or onto the practice field, he looks to achieve a performance result. The immediate experience is less important than the ultimate outcome. For this person, practice sessions are a means to an end: a record-setting performance or a physiological transformation such as weight-loss or an improved medical profile.

It's easy to see that individual exercisers have distinct preferences for classic or romantic points of view. In the stereotype, the romantic usually prefers dance, yoga, aikido and tai chi and wouldn't be caught dead with a clipboard or a heart rate monitor. He consistently looks for the experiential quality of movement and has no interest in keeping score or breaking records.

The classicist, on the other hand, tends to prefer weight lifting, running, swimming or any other activity that can be readily quantified and analyzed. He derives a sense of satisfaction from recording his performance and comparing it to previous efforts. For the classical extremist, the numbers may even become more important than the experience itself.

Naturally, these schools of thought tend to come into frequent conflict. Classicists consider romantics to be empty-headed dabblers who prefer mysticism to authentically challenging training. They see the romantic style as nothing more than a mystical veneer, something people do to avoid the genuine work that's necessary for physical transformation.

Romantics, on the other hand, view the classicists as insensitive automatons who bear a strong resemblance to the machines they work with such devoted labor. They may have impressive numbers, but if you take their clipboards away, they have nothing left.

The conflict goes deep. As Pirsig put it:

> To a romantic, the classic mode often appears dull, awkward and ugly. Everything's got to be measured and proved. Op-

pressive. Heavy. Endlessly grey. The death force. Within the classic mode, however, the romantic has some appearances of his own. Frivolous, irrational, erratic, untrustworthy, interested primarily in pleasure seeking. Shallow. Of no substance.

And when it gets really nasty, the romantic attempts to claim the mysto-spiritual high ground, usually talking about the power of intuition to trump the wicked and soulless machinery of the classicist. The classicist, for his part, lays claim to scientific certainty, backing it up with reams of data, footnotes, references and journal articles. For him, romantics are simply delusional.

TYRANNY OF THE CLASSICISTS

For my part, I've spent time in both camps. I've logged my mileage and tracked my numbers. I've filled out spreadsheets and graphed my performance. I've also had my share of romantic, passionate, whole-body experience. It's obvious that both approaches have their merits, but over time, I've come see some disturbing imbalances in our approach. That is, when it comes to matters of health, fitness and training, the classic mode is tyrannizing our perspective.

Everywhere we look in today's world, from the gym to the track to the clinic to the hospital, it's all about classical expertise, measurement and method. Logic and rationality have become the fundamental currency of the day. Professionalism is now linked directly to the classical point of view. We traffic almost exclusively in spreadsheets, forms, bullet points and checklists. We drive relentlessly towards measurement, research, data, proof, and statistics. Numbers rule our consciousness.

In the world of professionalized health, medicine and fitness, almost no one takes romantics seriously. Knowledge is only considered valid if it's measurable, trackable and independently verifiable. If you want some letters after your name, you'd better learn how to speak in numbers.

Not surprisingly, computers are driving this drift towards classical quantification. Classical ideas are easily digitized; it's a simple matter to track exercise on a spreadsheet. Sets, reps and mileage are easy to chart and easy to enter into a data base. The result looks professional. Authoritative. Credible.

Romantic experience, on the other hand, is messy and almost impossible to digitize. How do we squeeze passion and experience into bits and bytes? We can't. In fact, the moment we apply numbers and structure to romance, we kill the entire enterprise. (Just try tracking your lovemaking performance with a spreadsheet and see what it does for your relationship.) And so, in our devotion to computers, we simply choose to disregard the romantic point of view. If you can't digitize it, for all practical purposes, it doesn't even exist.

ROMANTIC PRIMATES

Classicists will argue long and hard for the merits of their position, but one fact trumps all their vocalizations—that is, when it comes to the animal world, romance is fundamental. Romance is primal. Romance lives in the deep structures of the primate brain, especially the limbic system. This circuitry is many millions of years older than the neocortex, the brain structure responsible for classical thinking.

Consider the non-human animals of the world, especially our closest primate relatives, the chimpanzees. These creatures have no interest in the classical mode of thought. They have no interest in systems, hierarchies, sequences, units, precision or quantification. They have no interest in sets or reps. They don't log mileage and they don't enter their performance on spreadsheets. And yet, their health and fitness is incredible.

I have been to Africa; I have seen the chimpanzees of Gombe, Tanzania. These animals are fit beyond belief. They are supremely strong, agile and endurant. But during my visit, I did not see a single chimpanzee with a clipboard. I did not see a single heart rate monitor, pedometer, spreadsheet or stopwatch. These animals did it all with gravity, vigorous movement, play and emotion.

A couple of simple thought experiments suggest that the classical approach is not at all necessary for health or fitness. Just imagine disease epidemic that somehow destroyed all human understanding of numbers. Or a hyper-infectious computer virus that wiped out every hard drive on earth. Could we still we still do physical education? Without numbers? Of course we could. All it would take is some romantic imagination. Get your tribe together and start moving. Make up some games and use whatever toys you've got on hand. Run some hills and climb some trees. Sing and dance. Pump some rocks and lift some logs. Chop wood and carry water. Play. Sure, you might not get your people to world-class status, but who cares? We've got a public health crisis on our hands; just getting people moving at all is success.

So maybe it's time to give the classical mode some time off; let the classicists have a vacation. Forget the data mongering, the performance tracking, the calorie-measuring, the sets, the reps and the mileage. Forget the spreadsheets, the online forms, the program administration and the credentials.

The message we need to take to heart is simple: Fall in love with movement and let it be contagious to those around you—it just might make a real difference.

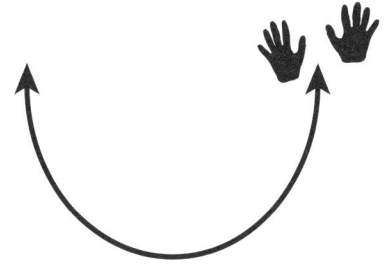

DEEP ARC
(GO LOW IN YOUR STANCE)

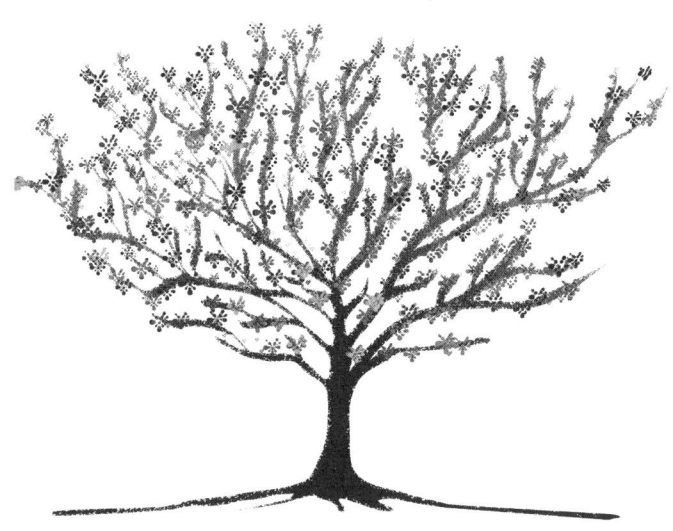

TAKE A CULTURE

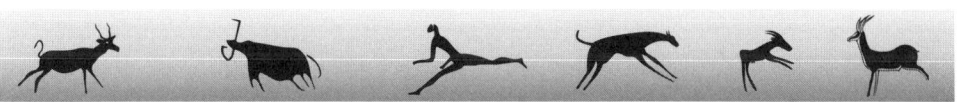

Change Your Body, Change the World

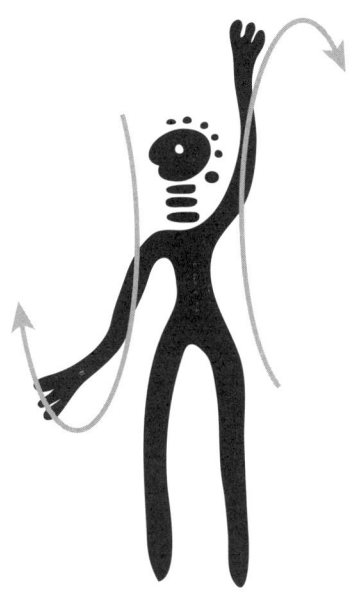

STANDING BACKSTROKE:
LONG STROKES, MANY STANCES

COGITO ERGO DUMB

> I am a brain, my dear Watson, and the rest of me is a mere appendage.
>
> Sherlock Holmes
> by Arthur Conan Doyle

> Wonder rather than doubt is the root of knowledge.
>
> Abraham Joshua Heschel

If you've ever enrolled at a major university, you've probably been drawn into that peculiar and often annoying game called "What's your major?"

It's the first week of freshman year and you're going through orientation. You've visited the bookstore, set up your class schedule and fixed up your dorm room just the way you like it. That evening you head to the cafeteria, load up your tray and make for the nearest table where you join a gaggle of new classmates. You introduce yourself and inevitably someone asks, "So, what's your major?"

At this point, you had better be ready with something impressive. Physics or philosophy would be good. Pre-something would also go over well: pre-law or pre-med would demonstrate your ambition as well as your high test scores. Engineering would be impressive, as would mathematics, chemistry, business or neuroscience. All of these disciplines are considered credible, worthy and compelling. All are proof of your substantial intelligence.

If you declare your interest in the humanities however, you're going to be skating on thin ice. Language, art and music are all acceptable as fields of study, but not nearly so impressive. ("Do you want fries with that?" will be the standard prediction of your employment potential.) Clearly, you're a couple of notches down the totem pole from the big dogs of academia, but you're still in the game. You're not going to be nominated for a Nobel prize anytime soon, but you'll probably get invited to a lot of parties all the same.

But whatever you do, make absolutely certain that you don't reveal that you're majoring in physical education. This will be a complete non-starter and will generate only an uneasy silence. Most of your friends will be surprised to hear that a PE major even exists; it's not even clear that you belong at a university in the first place. Inevitably, they'll picture you in a sweaty gym suit with a whistle hanging around your neck and a clipboard in your hand. You may have a great bod, but well, that's as far as it goes; for all practical purposes, you're dead from the neck up.

If you actually *are* majoring in physical education, be sure to dress it up in more acceptable clothing. Tell people that you're studying biomechanics, kinesiology or the anatomy of human movement. This will demonstrate your affiliation with physics and medicine, thus providing some measure of credibility. But whatever you do, don't mention PE.

ORIGINS

Everyone knows that PE is an academic backwater and a dead end, but why? Why is the study of human physicality so universally dissed? Why do we routinely demote our bodies to the lowest rung on the academic ladder? Do we really think so little of our physical selves?

I've pondered these questions for years and have become more perplexed at every turn. Aren't our bodies at the very core of who we are? Shouldn't our bodies have at least equal status with the arts and the sciences? Shouldn't the ability to manipulate our limbs have equal standing with our ability to manipulate abstract symbols? Where did this distorted bias come from?

After reviewing a host of possible explanations, I've come to the conclusion that much of the blame lies squarely with the perpetrator of the mind-body split, René Descartes.

Descartes, as you may recall, was a French philosopher, mathematician, scientist and writer in the early seventeenth century. He was a key figure in the scientific revolution and is sometimes described as the "Father of Modern Philosophy."

As a young man, Descartes undertook an epic quest for knowledge. He pondered the great questions of existence and resolved to doubt everything so as to get to the core of what was true and real. In the process he became a radical skeptic and even went so far as to doubt his own physical sensations.

After all, he famously mused, there might be an unseen evil demon at work, pumping false sensory information into his brain. How would he ever know? His brain could very well be floating in a vat of liquid, subject to the inputs of a mad operator with a hidden agenda; there was simply no way to tell.

So for Descartes, sensation was off the table as a reliable source of information. And since the body was not to be trusted, all that was left was the mind; this became his ultimate touchstone and identity. "I think, therefore I am" he famously declared. The body became irrelevant, except as a life support system for his prodigious feats of cognition.

Descartes' work was profoundly influential in his day and he soon became an icon of Western civilization. We have thoroughly incorporated his dualistic assumptions into our culture and our institutions. Today we honor the mind and neglect the body. We think, therefore we are. We move, therefore we are not.

And so, in spite of the fact that he's been dead for over 300 years, Descartes remains the biggest man on campus. When we sit around the table in the freshman cafeteria, we're playing out the implications of his mind-body dualism. We honor the students of the mind and devalue those who study the body. We accept a ranking system handed to us centuries ago, a system that now appears increasingly archaic, unhealthy and even absurd.

CONSEQUENCES

Unfortunately, there's a huge price to be paid for this mind-over-body value system. When we put the body at the bottom of our hierarchy, we should not be surprised to find a sedentary population completely out of touch with their physicality. We should not be surprised to find an epidemic of physical apathy and disease.

For better and for worse, the values of the university cascade downward through the rest of our educational system and out into the wider world: high schools mimic colleges, elementary schools mimic high schools. In the process, the body becomes devalued across the board. If resources are tight and something needs to be cut, PE is always the first to go. Test scores are vital we are told, but the body is expendable.

This ranking system plays out all across the health and medical landscape. Most of our modern lifestyle disease epidemics—heart disease, diabetes, depression and obesity—are highly preventable. And yet, we take almost no preemptive action. Instead, we wait for physical conditions to grow into full-blown diseases and then hand the problem off to the Cartesians at the top of the pyramid. When they succeed, we heap praise upon their heroic intelligence, but when they fail, we write it off as an intractable social problem.

The tragic irony is that Cartesian dualism has been soundly refuted by 100 years of research into mind-body relationships. We now know without question that the mind and body are intimately related. The conversation between tissue and cognition is complementary; the mind drives the body and the body drives the mind.

Antonio Damasio describes this integrated relationship in *Descartes' Error* (xvi–xvii):

> The human brain and the rest of the body constitute an indissociable organism, integrated by means of mutually interactive biochemical and neural regulatory circuits (including endocrine, immune, and autonomic neural components)...The organism interacts with the environment as an ensemble: the interaction is neither of the body alone nor of the brain alone...The physiological operation that we call mind is derived from the structural and functional ensemble rather than from the brain alone: mental phenomena can be fully understood only in the context of an organism's interacting in an environment.

Because of the tight interrelationship between mind and body, it is folly to put one above the other. Mind and body ought to be studied and enjoyed in equal proportion, as yin and yang. Rather than a totem pole with hard science on top and PE the bottom, we ought to imagine a circle with mind and body in intimate conversation with one another.

NO DUMB JOCKS

Our conventional academic hierarchy makes even less sense now that the "dumb jock" myth is finally being laid to rest. Hundreds of research studies have proven beyond question that vigorous physical movement is good for the brain and in turn, intelligence. Far from being dumb, people who move their bodies do better across a wide span of cognitive challenges. Movement makes us smarter.

Some will continue to cling to "dumb jock" mythology of course, but the prejudice is getting weaker every day. We now know that physical movement promotes neurogenesis, the birth of new brain cells, and synaptogenesis, the growth of neural connections. Vigorous movement also promotes the production of BDNF (brain derived neurotrophic factor), sometimes described as "miracle grow for the brain." Vigorous movement also reduces the corrosive effects of stress hormones, which in turn preserves the function of the hippocampus, the brain's essential memory center.

So, far from being dumb, it's beginning to appear that, all other things being equal, jocks actually have a mental edge over their sedentary counterparts. Eventually, we will be forced to readjust our stereotypes.

ALTERNATIVE PHILOSOPHIES

As I ponder the long reach of Cartesian dualism and its pathological effects on human health, I often wonder how different our world would be if Descartes had been an athlete, a dancer or a martial artist. Instead of doubting his senses, he would have learned to trust and sharpen them. His attention would have gone out into the world and, in turn, his philosophical writings would have been more integrative. He would have emphasized relationship, continuity and connection.

And so I imagine myself as a coach to the young René, getting him out of his office and out onto the land. I'd have him run the trails and climb the mountains of Europe. I'd teach him to develop and trust his sensory capabilities. I'd give him lots of multi-plane movement to stimulate fresh connections in his nervous system. I'd drag him out of the library and into the open air. I'd help him see the magic of human physicality.

It was not inevitable that Descartes would mistrust the body and choose to identify with the mind. Given a different life experience or a creative coach, he might have come to entirely different conclusions: "I feel, therefore I am," (Accipio ergo sum.) "I wonder, therefore I am," (Admiror ergo sum.) "I dance, therefore I am," (Chorea ergo sum.) "I play, therefore I am." (Adludo ergo sum.) "I move, therefore I am," (Agilis ergo sum.) "I create, therefore I am," (Aedifico ergo sum.) or "I love, therefore I am. (Amo ergo sum.)

I AM PHYSICAL, THEREFORE I AM

So, maybe it's time for another look at "What's your major?" Instead of resigning ourselves to a seat at the back of the academic bus, perhaps it's time to stand up for the human body and an integrative course of study. Maybe it's time to challenge the status quo and insist on having a voice in the conversation. Ask the Cartesians how their massive brains are going to function without a healthy, active body. If they give you an evasive, abstracted reply, drag them away from their computers and get them out into the open air. Invite them to kick off their shoes and get back into their bodies. Give them some vigorous movement and then have another conversation. Chances are, their thoughts will become a touch more integrated and comprehensible.

And who knows? They might even change majors.

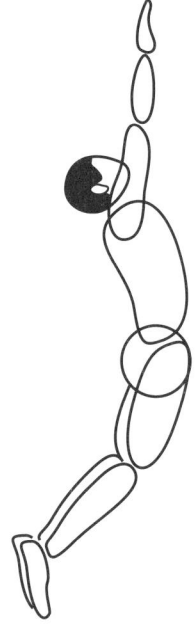

PATHOLOGY ON PARADE

For those who are awake the cosmos is one and common, but those who sleep turn away each into a private world.

Heraclitus

In the spring of 2009, the Exuberant Animal tribe was invited to give a presentation at the Arnold Active Aging Festival in Columbus, Ohio. (That's Arnold, as in Schwarzenegger.) At the time, it seemed like a good idea. We were delighted to share our philosophy of play-based fitness and health promotion with the senior community. We soon discovered however, that the Active Aging event was actually a side-show to a mega-spectacle at the convention center next door: the Arnold Bodybuilding Festival.

The bodybuilding event itself was prodigious in every dimension. Everywhere we looked we saw extremity, enormity and excess; everything was huge, loud and in your face. The displays were incredible statements in their own right, but it was the bodies that really stopped us in our tracks. Everywhere we looked we saw immense, distorted, alien bodies of preposterous proportion—muscle and silicone as far as the eye could see.

The pathos of the event was clearly expressed in the advertisements for various products, mostly supplements. Company names included "Brutal," "Armageddon," "House of Pain," "Punishment Athletics," "Body Fortress," ("Your body, your fortress.") "Beast," "Affliction," and our personal favorite, "Biohazard Nutrition." Supplement brands included: "Absolute Domination," "Dark Rage," "Beyond Extreme," "Monster Milk," "Respect," "Retaliate," "Jet Fuel," "Redline," "Myo Shock," "Nightmare" and "WAR" ("Workout Anabolic Response") We were welcomed with t-shirts telling us to "Go heavy or go home," "Shut the fuck up and train," "Throw up" and "Go away."

We didn't know whether to laugh, cry or flee for our lives. Our emotions swung from abhorrence and disgust to dismay and morbid fascination. One of our trainers described the experience as "watching our culture circling the drain." After leaving the convention hall, he spoke for all of us when he said simply, "I feel diseased."

WHAT'S HEALTH GOT TO DO WITH IT?

The convention was billed as a "health and fitness event," but clearly health had nothing whatsoever to do with it. Most participants were in obvious partnership with the biochemical devil, mortgaging their futures for short-term muscular development.

In essence, this event resembled nothing so much as a vast chemistry experiment: take immense quantities of anabolic substances, add prodigious amounts of brute physical labor and presto—spectacular muscular development! If you wanted, you could reproduce the whole thing in a laboratory.

Only the most naïve observer would have wondered about steroid use in this population. Some things are simply obvious. No amount of natural training would produce such grotesque physical development. The tissue that we observed was clearly synthetic and freakishly unnatural. As one observer put it, "If cannibalism were legal, you wouldn't want to put any of these people on the barbecue."

There was no ambiguity about the ultimate purpose of this event. Obviously, the primary objective was to promote the appearance and experience of individual human bodies. As such, this event was poised at the cutting edge of the "me industry."

Bodybuilders are the most obvious players in this industry, but they are by no means the only ones. The "me industry" is an immense, culture-wide force that includes most health, fitness and lifestyle magazines, TV shows, books and DVDs, as well as many gyms, spas and salons. In addition to an obsessive focus on muscle and weight loss, it also includes athletic achievement, skin care, fashion and personal possession. In this industry, attention is centered exclusively on the individual and the individual's body. It's all about *your* abs or *my* butt. It's all about *your* weight loss or *my* athletic performance. It's all about *your* hair or *my* skin. It's never about *our* community or *our* predicament.

DARK ART

The primary themes of the day were pain, suffering, isolation and darkness; there were no life-affirming messages anywhere. We saw no expressions of joy, celebration or exuberance, although there was plenty of self-abuse and punishment. Beat your body into submission. Pain is the path to achievement and spectacular mass. Happiness is for pussies and skinny people. Only through brutal, self-inflicted punishment can one gain mastery over tissue and life. As the Body Force tagline puts it so clearly, "The best bodies are built by force."

Supplement companies went to great lengths to demonstrate their commitment to intentional suffering, constructing fully-enclosed chain-link training areas decorated in an urban-industrial motif, complete with black 55-gallon steel drums. These cages were intentionally designed to focus the pain and isolation as intensively as possible.

There was nothing ambiguous about it; these enclosures featured caged human animals doing battle with heavy iron. Lifters embraced their condition and reveled in its meaning, but we were stunned. It was inconceivable to us that a person would build a cage and inhabit it voluntarily. After all, the normal animal response to captivity is escape. No wild animal would ever voluntarily inhabit such a cage, much less build one for the express purpose of locking itself up.

IS THE UNIVERSE FRIENDLY?

As we wandered the convention hall, each of us was given to wonder: What set of circumstances would lead people to such extremity? What kind of life would produce such a pathological orientation to the body and the world?

We can only imagine the original cause of such dysfunction, but one thing seemed certain. These individuals must have, at some point in their lives, considered Einstein's famous question and concluded—consciously or otherwise—that no, the universe is *not* friendly.

And of course, when you live in an unfriendly world, you've got to do everything possible to secure your position. Threats are everywhere, options are limited, possibilities few, people are treacherous, relationships are ambiguous, security is fleeting.

If this is your worldview, it makes sense to seek out power and control by any means possible. Intimidate your adversaries with outrageous appearance, buy them off with wealth, overcome them with skill or intimidate them with weapons. Naturally, this orientation becomes a vicious circle of self-fulfillment: the more we defend, the more hostile the world becomes.

And so we see a dark synergy of disciplines and practices, bound together by fear and insecurity. Call it "the insecurity-industrial complex" if you will—this network includes bodybuilding, mixed martial arts, ultimate fighting, military combat, weapons and, of course, porno. When we encounter one of these practices, we're sure to find the others lurking nearby.

And so it seemed somehow fitting that the US Army would have a display booth of its own featuring a state-of-the-art interactive video game called "Door Gunner." A replica assault rifle was mounted on a tripod, poised to take aim at the wide-screen display and a pair of friendly young soldiers, dressed in desert camo, invited visitors to take a turn on the weapon. As the action rolled, we watched transfixed as an incredibly realistic aerial scene unfolded. Suddenly we were flying over a Middle Eastern city, watching as our "gunner" picked off people in the streets. The action was utterly convincing. Most visitors seemed to find it entertaining and instructive, but we were horrified.

AS THE WORLD BURNS

Outside the convention hall, environmental reality was still in full swing. Climate was still warming and destabilizing at a frightening rate and natural systems were threatening to crash in every direction. But inside, planetary reality was held at bay. We observed no hint of ecological or social consciousness on any level. On the contrary, we witnessed spectacular, extravagant waste in a variety of forms: wasted resources, wasted potential, wasted intelligence and of course, wasted health.

We could only wonder: given our planetary predicament, how could anyone justify this lifestyle? How much carbon was pumped into the atmosphere to make this event possible? How much plastic was produced and discarded? How much fresh water was wasted in chemical processing? How many animals were slaughtered to produce the mountains of protein that were being consumed in such radical excess? We could only wonder how this spectacle would appear to the impoverished citizens of our planet, the billion or so people who scrape and scavenge each day for mere subsistence.

THE BODY IS A MIRROR

I have long believed that the human body is a reflection of culture, a mirror that allows us to see who we are and how we live in the world. So the question arises: what does the increasing popularity of extreme bodybuilding tell us about who we are as a society?

It tells us that we are insecure and fearful. It tells us that we are terrified of our predicament. We feel powerless. We feel that we lack control.

Of course, bodybuilding is an easy target; the practice public and the dysfunction is obvious. But we can be sure that our culture is home to other forms of fear-based extremism that are less visible to our eyes. After all, bodybuilders can claim no monopoly on obsessive-compulsive behavior.

And so we are forced to ask some hard questions: How is this form of obsession different from any other? Is the bodybuilder any different from the corporate workaholic? The triathlete? The aspiring Olympian? What do we expect in a culture that rewards extremity of all varieties? What do we expect in a culture that glorifies the individual over community?

There should be no surprise here. The bodybuilding sub-culture is the logical outcome of a larger culture in which extremity is not only tolerated, but celebrated. And in this sense, the problem doesn't lie within the bodybuilding culture itself; the problem lies with us. Of course the bodybuilding culture is diseased. But if bodybuilders are out of balance, so too is anyone who devotes every waking moment to a physical specialty or monomaniacal pursuit: the ultramarathoners, the fanatical mountain climbers and the yoga practitioners who spend decades twisting their bodies into impossible poses. Bodybuilders have no monopoly on physical extremism or lifestyle dysfunction.

WHERE'S THE HEALTH?

In the end, the Arnold festival experience brought me to a higher level of confusion. For years I have agonized over the state of the modern human body, especially our epidemic of sedentary living and physical apathy. But here I observed something altogether different. The bodybuilders weren't sedentary and they obviously weren't obese, but they certainly weren't healthy.

As I stepped outside the convention center, I was struck by the incredible contrast. Hundreds of "normal," obese Americans walked by, their massive, diabetic bodies struggling to make the trip from car to restaurant. Suddenly I began to feel like Diogenes walking the streets with a lamp on a dark night. But instead of looking for one honest man, I was looking for one truly healthy man or woman.

Or better yet, a healthy culture.

My search continues…

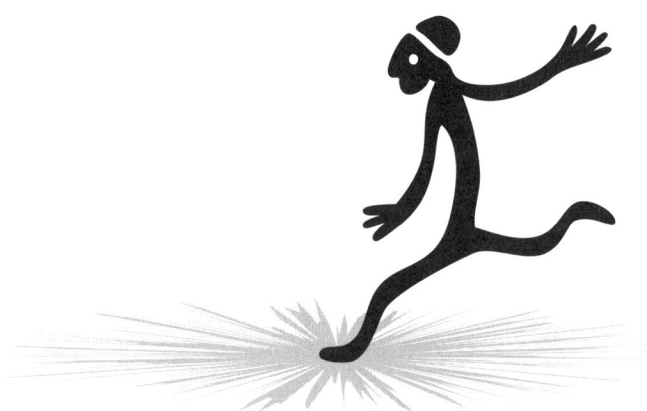

STEP-N-STOP:
STICK THE LANDING WITH PERFECT BALANCE

I KNOW IT WHEN I SEE IT

> A superstimulus or superreleaser is an exaggerated version of a stimulus to which there is an existing response tendency…
>
> Wikipedia

People say that I have a dirty mind and I guess they must be right. You see, I've been thinking a lot about pornography lately. Not just the plastic-wrapped, behind-the-counter skin mags, but all kinds of smut. Conventional porn, alternative porn, health and fitness porn, food porn, marketing porn—I've been meditating on all of it. And now, after an intensive period of dedicated study, I've come to the realization that porn may have some problems.

Now please be advised that I have nothing against sex. Nor do I have a problem with robust, wild sex or even sex in public. And as for sex with animals, well, that's what it's all about, right? Animals have been having wild sex in public for something like 500 million years, ever since the Cambrian explosion. And as for us, sex with humans is profoundly natural and normal; people really ought to be doing more of it.

So what's the problem? Well, the popular definition of pornography focuses on sexual imagery, "dirty" pictures of naked people doing "nasty" things related to copulation. But I take a broader view. The way I see it, pornography is anything that takes us directly from impulse to gratification. The thing about porn is that it gets directly to the point. It's blatant, abrupt and completely unambiguous. There's no subtlety, no nuance, no romance, no seduction, no warm-up, no anticipation, no nurturing of the appetite. It drops you directly into a fantasy realm and pumps you to exhaustion.

SUPERNORMAL STIMULATION

Not only does porno deliver, it delivers sensations, ideas and imagery that are richer and more robust than would normally occur in real life; it's reality-plus. Comedian Richard Jeni reminds us of this fact when he describes pornographic movies as "things that will never happen to you in your lifetime." For many of us, porn is sort of like regular sex, only a whole lot better. The people are more attractive, more energetic and more open-minded, not to mention more endurant and more orgasmic than you or I will ever be. (When was the last time you had wild group sex in the photocopy room of your office?)

This is precisely the point that Deidre Barrett brings to light in her recent book *Waistland: The (R)Evolutionary Science Behind Our Weight and Fitness Crisis*. For Barrett, the crucial factor in our health and fitness predicament is the disruption of normal behavior by "supernormal stimuli." This term is borrowed from the study of animal behavior (ethology) and refers to artificial objects that appeal to our instincts more strongly than the natural foods or activities for which those instincts originally evolved. Barrett believes that because of these supernormal stimuli, we eat far more than we would otherwise eat and even worse, we are drawn to over-eat the wrong kind of things.

The study of hyper-stimulation started with ethologist Niko Tinbergen, winner of the 1973 Nobel prize in biology for his research on instinctive behavior in animals. Tinbergen devised a series of dummy objects, specifically designed to surpass the power of a natural stimulus. For example, he found that many bird species preferred plaster eggs that were larger than their own and that were decorated with exaggerated colors or markings. Some species will even ignore their own eggs in favor of over-sized fakes. Songbirds will abandon their own pale blue eggs to mount a huge day-glow dummy egg. When a greylag goose is given the choice between its own egg and a volleyball, it chooses to sit on the volleyball.

GOING SUPERNORMAL

So what happens when you put an animal into a world of supernormal stimuli, a pornosphere if you will? Obviously, you're going to wind up with a seriously distracted animal, one that behaves in ways that are inconsistent with that animal's natural history. As Barrett puts it, supernormal stimuli "hijack our natural instincts." Supernormal stimuli generate excitement, distraction and disordered attention. They also lead to diminished interest in normal stimuli. After all, once you've eaten a sugary, salty, artificially flavored food product, who wants to go back to eating boring, natural, unadulterated food? Once you've sat on a volleyball, who wants to sit on a regular egg? Once you've had a faux-sex experience with porn star, who wants to go back to sleeping with regular people?

For Barrett, supernormal stimuli can also lead to addiction. "Heroin and high-fructose corn syrup are reinforcing because they're intensified versions of natural endorphins and natural glucose levels respectively." Ultimately, continuous exposure to supernormal stimuli leads us towards aberrant, unnatural behaviors. Sometimes these behaviors are spectacularly perverse, other times they are subtle variations on normal lifestyle. In either case, slight preferences for the supernormal, exercised over years and decades, can add up to some serious health consequences. Just ask a type-2 diabetic.

FAST FOOD SMUT

At this point, we need to remember that our baseline for normal sensory stimulation is our Paleolithic grassland experience: the semi-wooded mosaic habitat of the ancient past. If you lived in such a world, you'd find that most stimuli were subtle: colors were generally muted earth tones, shapes were soft, sounds were quiet, and with the exception of occasional predator attacks, events moved slowly.

In contrast, today's fast-food stimuli screams at us with the promise of instant gratification, often in the form of super-refined salt and sugar, all promoted with high-contrast colors and imagery. There's no nurturing of the appetite, no time-consuming hunting or gathering, no careful preparation, no fretting over ingredients. Just a direct path from impulse to gratification. No anticipation, no process, just an instant product that tastes better than anything you'd ever find on the grassland. No wonder we're so distracted.

In fact, today's nutritional stimulation is thousands of times more powerful than what would have occurred on the grassland. Not only are our "foods" artificially enhanced for maximum flavor, they surround us wherever we go; no walking or searching is required. Even worse, our media reminds us constantly that such flavor sensations are just a click or a call away. A hunter-gatherer might walk half a day to get a few bittersweet berries off a bush, but the modern urbanite can secure an enormous bag of far sweeter treats, just by pushing a few buttons or pointing his car in the right direction. Thus, an epidemic of obesity, diabetes and heart disease.

THE GOLDEN AGE OF PORN

It's not just food porn that leads us astray. Once we start to think in terms of supernormal stimuli, we begin to see it everywhere. For example, the fitness industry is thick with porn. Not only does it overlap strongly with sex porn, it also deceives us with a promise of instant fitness. In fact, every promise of "get fit quick" or "get rich quick" is porn, pure and simple. The ubiquitous "before and after" photo spread is just as pornographic as the photo-manipulated picture of McFood on the passing 18-wheeler, just as pornographic as the skin mags behind the counter at the mini-mart. Anyone who promises instant results is by definition a pornographer.

In the wide world of sports, the highlight clip is also porn. No longer is there any need to sit through a tedious stretch of first quarter maneuvering, routine jump shots, three-yard runs or base hits. Being a fan no longer means being a student of the game. Instead, we flit from one sporting titillation to the next, remote control in hand, alert for the most spectacular, arousing, athletic-erotic moments. By comparison, watching an entire game seems torturously dull. We want a sporting climax and we want it now.

Pornographic images even distort our relationship with the natural world. One environmental writer has referred to glossy telephoto images of wild animals as "eco-porn." His point is that these images, appealing as they might be, completely misrepresent the reality of the natural world. Spend too much time flipping though popular nature magazines and you'll come to expect that lions, tigers and bears are standing shoulder to shoulder in every forest, swamp and alpine meadow. In fact, sightings of these creatures are rare and require tremendous patience. People who are raised on eco-porn are often frustrated when they visit wild areas; they expect to see large animals everywhere, hunting and humping in every direction. Disappointed, they return to their living rooms where they can see some "real" action on TV. In contrast, nature is just too dull to bother with.

THE USE AND ABUSE OF PORN

Moralists like to make blanket condemnations of skin porn and they'd probably make similar condemnations of all supernormal stimuli. They might even suggest that we practice a kind of sensory chastity, limiting our exposure to all-natural sensations: the primal colors, sounds, textures and odors that our bodies have been exposed to for millions of years.

The moralists might make a good case, but the fact remains that supernormal sensations can have legitimate, healthy uses, especially when they stimulate our creativity. Bright colors and novel sounds can spark new art forms and valuable expressions. Modern art and electronic music are supernormal, but they have also given us some invaluable contributions.

In the right circumstances, supernormal stimuli can provoke new ideas and innovation. Such stimuli might even spark neurological development, neurogenesis and synaptic connectivity. Not surprisingly, artists of all types are attracted to novel stimuli and make good use of it. The same is probably true for skin-porn itself, by the way. In the right hands and at the right moment, vivid sexual imagery might be the ideal stimulus for creative sensual pleasure and adventurous lovemaking.

By itself and in small doses, porn is probably harmless. Soft food porn, soft fitness porn, soft skin porn: in the right circumstance, all of these forms might very well enrich our lives. A few titillations, a little extra excitement, some quick stimulation keeps life interesting and can even relieve the tedium that many of us are forced to endure each day.

But today, porn is everywhere and a lot of it is truly hard core, in-your-face, round-the-clock smut. Modern media has given us a pornosphere in which supernormal stimuli are virtually impossible to ignore. And being ubiquitous, porn now threatens to undermine our collective attention, our happiness and our health.

THE ANTIDOTE

Clearly, we need some kind of antidote to the modern porn glut, some means of insulating our psyches from hypersensory stimulation. Herein lies the crux of the problem: the human brain is extremely vulnerable to the supernormal stimuli cooked up by today's pornographers. In fact, this is their core objective: to burrow directly into the deepest levels of the human brain and manipulate our emotional responses. Pornographers want our money of course, but first they need to control our minds.

The antidote to this pornographic marketing crusade lies in the prefrontal cortex, a brain structure that can regulate and dampen impulsive, emotional responses. The prefrontal cortex acts as a counterweight to the powerful, surging desires of the limbic system, the paleo-mammalian brain.

Unfortunately, the prefrontal cortex doesn't fully mature until the mid-20's, which helps explain why young people are more vulnerable to all kinds of supernormal imagery and sensation. And to make matters worse, the prefrontal cortex is vulnerable to the effects of stress. Glucocorticoids (stress hormones) not only damage neurons in the hippocampus (a vital memory center), they also degrade the capabilities of the prefrontal cortex. Thus, the more stressed you get, the more susceptible you become to impulse, the more vulnerable you become to porn.

Consequently, stress-reducing practices are essential. If you want to protect yourself from the excesses of pornographic stimuli, it makes sense to pamper yourself with relaxation and rejuvenation. Take care of your brain and you'll be in a better position to take care of your body.

PORNO-PROOFING

For my part, I've always been an advocate of natural living and trusted my body to make good choices instinctively. But now I'm beginning to see the folly of my ways. In a porno-saturated world, we can no longer trust our bodies to make wise choices. There are simply too many pathological forces out there competing for our attention and distorting our behavior. Given free reign to act on impulse, our bodies will go for the porn every time. Without some countervailing force, we eventually become pornovores.

So, we need to guard our experience, intentionally and consciously. As Barrett puts it, we need to "ignore instinctual signals and listen to our intellect." This, I'm sad to say, requires a measure of discipline, patience and lifestyle ritual.

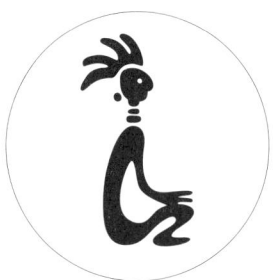

The good news is that there are many ways to develop prefrontal control. Almost any discipline should work, whether it be athletics, music, writing or craft. All skill development requires prefrontal regulation and thus confers some immunity to porn. But of all the porno-proofing methods available to us, meditation seems to offer the greatest promise. After all, if you can sit still in one place for a few minutes each day, watching your breath with focused attention, observing your own thoughts without reacting to them, you will develop a much stronger prefrontal muscle for fending off the flood of pornographic sensation that will surely come your way. It's definitely worth a try.

While we're at it, we might try adjusting our values: Instead of falling victim to the pornographic speed machine, we might try slowing down. Honor desire, build hunger and take pleasure in process. Appreciate the romance, the seduction, the warm up, the pre-season. The slow road to gratification may feel alien and it's definitely counter-cultural, but it's the healthiest path for our bodies and our spirits. Slow Food, Slow Fitness, Slow Sex, Slow Success. Stretch out your experience and enjoy the path.

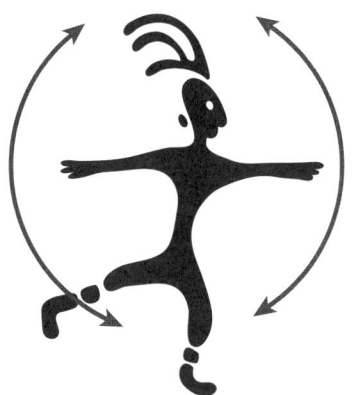

STANDING ARM SWINGS: ALL STANCES

DOJO RULES

Only one who devotes himself to a cause with his whole strength and soul can be a true master. For this reason mastery demands all of a person.

>Albert Einstein

The uncommitted life isn't worth living.

>Marshall Fishwick

In the world of martial art, everyone likes to brag about how great their sensei is, or was: "My sensei could break 10 bricks!" "Yeah, well my sensei could catch arrows in flight!" "Yeah, well my sensei can beat up your sensei!" And on it goes, everyone boasting about the powers of his or her master teacher.

Well it's different for me. You see, my sensei was a real bonehead. He didn't know anything about training, exercise or physical education. He knew how to read, but didn't. He didn't go to seminars and he didn't keep up with the latest research, recommendations and standards.

To make matters worse, he didn't know anything about exercise science. He didn't know the origins and insertions of the muscles. He didn't know the difference between a tendon and a ligament. He didn't know any biomechanics or kinesiology. He didn't know anything about nutrition or proper hydration. He wasn't certified in CPR or first aid. He didn't know how to calculate a target heart rate or how to periodize a training program. He didn't know the proper form for a squat and he didn't know how to program a treadmill or Stairmaster. He didn't know anything about cross-training, intervals or Pilates. And to top it all off, he didn't know anything about pedagogy or the philosophy of education; I can guarantee that he'd never heard of John Dewey, William James or Jean Piaget.

And finally, to make matters worse, he had no letters after his name. No MA, PhD, MD, DC, PT, RN, CSCS, ATC, or LMT. Just a name. In fact, he only had one "credential" —a faded cotton belt that wrapped around his training uniform. Once black, it was so worn and abraded that appeared almost completely white. If you didn't know who he was, you might well have mistaken him for a garden-variety white belt. Until he started moving, that is.

Given the magnitude of my sensei's ignorance, one might suppose that his dojo was an abject failure, that his students failed to progress, that they languished in atrophy, frustration and ill-health. We might imagine that they endured long hours of pointless, injury-promoting exercise, eventually dropping out to become public health statistics.

But that's not how it went. My sensei got spectacular and enduring results. He was a force of nature: powerful, physically educated and dedicated to the process and his students. His dojo was simple, low-budget and profoundly successful. It touched many lives and produced a long string of graduates, each with an increased respect for self, others and the training process. These people became healthier, happier and more successful. During my apprenticeship, I saw incredible physical transformations. Slow, awkward bodies walked in, and a few years later, walked out lean, agile and proud. No modern technology or methods required, just gobs and gobs of sincere and consistent participation. The secret formula, as sensei so often put it, was "time on the mat."

THE FORMULA

My sensei's success was based, not any institutionalized program of standards and administration, but on the intangibles that have always contributed to success. He was in love with the process and in love with the art. He was devoted to his students. He took immense pride in his work. He went out on the mat and taught classes even on those nights when he felt terrible, even when his life wasn't working so well. When he stepped into the dojo, he gave it everything he had.

For my sensei, the key to success was full participation and immersion in the process; there was simply no room for dabbling or drop-ins. All students were required to keep their commitments and train hard. This expectation applied across the board, no exceptions.

Sensei ran his dojo with a simple set of rules that had been passed down to him during the course of his training, thus preserving an ancient tradition. These rules were implicit to the everyday operation of the dojo and applied equally to everyone. Whether explicit or implicit, most successful dojos and organizations follow a similar set of guidelines:

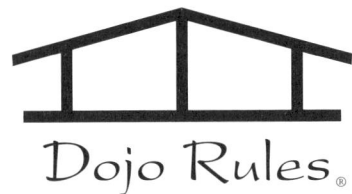

- Show respect for people, process and place.
- Exercise radical responsibility: own your circumstances.
- Seek balance, harmony and integration.
- Balance gravity and levity with serious play.
- Focus attention and presence. Be here now.
- Participate fully with end-to-end commitment.
- Everyone trains with everyone.
- Come with an empty cup, ready to learn.
- Seek transformation and excellence.
- Save face: praise in public, punish in private.
- Walk your talk: seek personal integration.
- Develop a growth orientation: focus on the process.

SACRED SPACE AND TIME

Intuitively, my sensei understood that full participation was the key ingredient to success. This same principle holds true by the way, for *any* educational process or transformative enterprise whether it be professional development, athletics, physical education, music, dance, art, relationships or scholarship. If it's worth doing at all, it's worth showing up on time and staying for the duration. Learning requires commitment; we can be sure there were no drop-in classes at the Shaolin temple. Thus the importance of firewalls and boundaries: this time and this space are sacred.

Unfortunately, our culture is moving in precisely the opposite direction. Today we actively promote a style of living that is designed for convenience, not substance. Nothing's important and nothing's worth prioritizing. It's all browsing, all dabbling, all shopping. Everyone's on the run, too busy to live and too busy to learn.

Advertisers drive this culture by catering to the customer's every desire. The market jumps at the chance to cater to our every whim, no matter how trivial. At the same time, it leans away from any enterprise that requires substantial levels of time, investment or commitment. The marketer's motto for maximizing sales: "Make it as easy as possible."

Which is precisely the problem. When it comes to making substantive changes to minds, bodies or lives, easy doesn't work. Easy doesn't transform. All easy does is grease the path from impulse to a shallow gratification. Easy doesn't save time; easy is a waste of time.

This is why our modern convenience culture fails so spectacularly. By maximizing ease, it simultaneously minimizes commitment. By minimizing commitment, it strips away meaning. And by stripping away meaning, it trivializes everything it touches.

Dabbling sets us up for failure because it allows us an easy exit in times of challenge. The dabbler develops a habit of partial engagement and positions himself for quick and easy retreat. Then, when the process becomes difficult or uncomfortable, he makes the quick exit. Those who drop in are quick to drop out.

A CULTURE OF COMMITMENT

If we're really, truly serious about transforming our bodies and public health, we're going to have to stop catering to the dabblers and start developing sacred times and spaces with an ethic of full participation. We're going to have to require a culture of commitment and an authentic sense of engagement, risk and immersion.

This means holding the line and protecting our most important times and spaces from distraction, intrusion and trivialization. No matter whether we're running a business, a school or a dojo, the same principles of participation and integrity apply. We're doing real and important work here and it's essential that we protect it and keep it whole.

My sensei ran his dojo for a couple of decades, a pretty good run by martial art standards. In the process, he turned out dozens of black belts and hundreds of brown belts. He gave health, fitness and pride to thousands of people. He created an environment that encouraged growth and challenged students to create their own transformations of mind, body and spirit.

In the end, his limited knowledge of exercise science and educational pedagogy made not one whit of difference. Sure, if he had known a bit more about muscle physiology, we might not have pulled so many hamstrings, but what of it? For what my sensei accomplished, I'll take the hamstring pulls any day.

You see, my sensei was great.

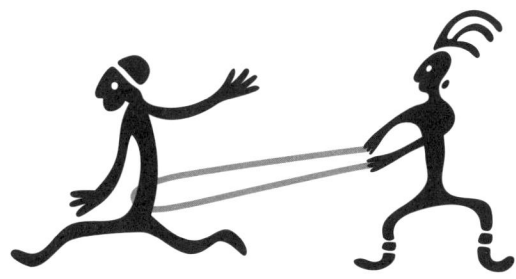

PARTNER-RESIST:
SLOW YOUR PARTNER DOWN WITH SMOOTH RESISTANCE
FORWARD, LATERAL AND ZIG-ZAGS

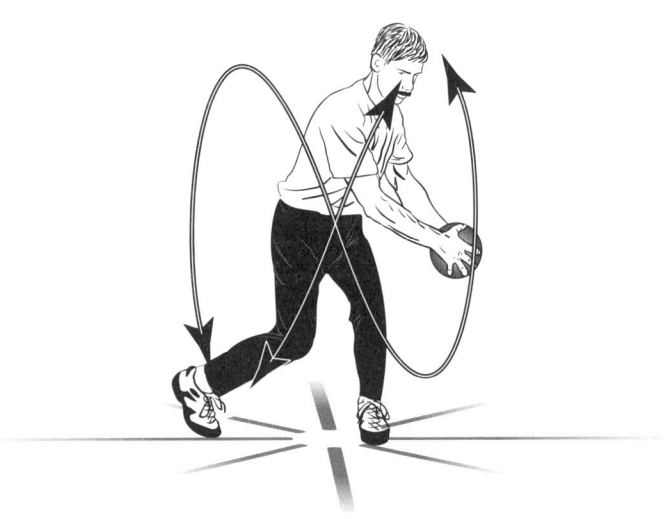

INTEGRATED, WHOLE-BODY 8'S WITH THE MED BALL:
ENGAGE BUTT, HIPS AND CORE

ROBOTS ARE FROM MARS, HUMANS ARE FROM EARTH

> It is only insofar as we renounce the world as its lovers that we can conquer it as its technicians. But this division in the soul is fatal to what is best in man...The power conferred by science as a technique is only obtainable by something analogous to the worship of Satan, that is to say, by the renunciation of love...The scientific society in its pure form...is incompatible with the pursuit of truth, with love, with art, with spontaneous delight, with every ideal that men have hitherto cherished.
>
> Bertrand Russell

When I was an undergrad, I was in way over my head. I was a jock, admitted to the university by virtue of my ability to chase a yellow rubber ball around a swimming pool. I had no idea how to take notes, study for exams or organize my classes. To me, the university was an utterly foreign land; I had no map, no phrase book and no guide.

I sat in the back row of my lecture classes, incapacitated by my ignorance and the sheer incomprehensibility of what I was hearing. The language sounded like English, but I couldn't understand a word of it. I managed to bluff my way through exams by sheer force of memory, but despite my efforts, I remained lost in the woods.

As the semesters passed, I became increasingly distressed, especially with a curious reference I heard almost every day. Inexplicably, most of my professors seemed to be fascinated with some guy from Mars. And it wasn't just astronomy class either; almost every professor made reference to this mysterious, cosmic individual. Biology, physiology, social science, geology, it didn't matter—everyone was talking about the Martian. Each professor would introduce a challenging subject, address it from a couple of perspectives and then tell us what the Man from Mars would think about it.

This confused me to no end. I knew where Mars was, more or less, and I could even imagine myself standing on that distant planet, looking back at Earth and taking a long view of its biology and the behavior of its inhabitants. But still, I had no idea why the Man from Mars was so important. Why did so many of my professors refer to him and defer to him? And why did they never speak of a "Man from Earth" or a "Woman from Earth" for that matter? Clearly, something fishy was going on.

It took me a couple of decades to sort it all out, but I finally came to understand why the Man from Mars was held in such great esteem. The problem began back in the Renaissance, when natural philosophers, now known as scientists, first began to appreciate the human capacity for self-delusion. A string of realizations and discoveries was wreaking havoc with our common perceptions: It looks like the Sun goes around the Earth, but it doesn't. It feels like our conscious minds are in charge of our lives and our bodies, but they aren't. It appears that we are fundamentally different from all the other animals around us, but we aren't. Copernicus, Freud and Darwin exposed our faulty reasoning and showed us just how mistaken our perceptions can be.

And that was just the beginning. In the 20th century, we discovered the power of the placebo effect, the psychosocial influences of "groupthink" and the almost limitless ways in which we can trick ourselves through social pressure, desire and misplaced attention. We began to realize that human beings have an enormous capacity for self-deception and outright delusion. Consequently, it's easy for our inquiries to go astray.

So, to protect ourselves from illusion and error, we conjured up the Man from Mars, a symbol of remote objectivity, a philosophical antidote to self-delusion. My professors believed that, if we could simply adopt this remote and objective view, we would see the world as it truly is. Thus, by the time I arrived at the university, the Man from Mars was the true big man on campus.

MARTIAN CULTURE

Of course, the Man from Mars isn't really a man at all, or a woman, or even a whole animal for that matter. He's just a disembodied, abstracted eyeball, a point of view floating in space. No flesh to distract him, no hormones or neuropeptides to sway his judgment or bias his view. He's objective, rational, and completely without emotion.

Naturally, this dispassionate perspective reveals itself in Martian behavior, if we can call it that. You see, nobody plays on Mars. Nobody dances, celebrates or moves their bodies. Nobody does art. Nobody takes recess or goes on vacation. Nobody plays music, makes love or writes poetry. All the Martians do is observe, gather data, organize their references and write journal articles. It's all very sterile. It's all very dead. And it isn't even close to being healthy.

I am not the first to make such observations about the Man from Mars and his abstracted point of view. In his landmark 1981 book, *The Reenchantment of the World*, historian Morris Berman described two basic styles of knowing: participating and non-participating consciousness. The difference between these two strategies is simple: while the Man from Earth holds an integrated view of himself in the world, the Man from Mars intentionally casts himself as an outsider, an extraterrestrial. The Man from Earth lives inside his experience; the Man from Mars steps outside, way outside.

According to Berman, non-participating consciousness is "that state of mind in which one knows phenomena precisely in the act of distancing oneself from them." Knowledge of nature comes about, not by way of experience and contact via the body, but by separation. In other words, "scientific consciousness is alienated consciousness: there is no ecstatic merger with nature, but rather total separation from it." This has become the Prime Directive of modern academics and administration: Look all you like, but whatever you do, don't touch.

THE HUMAN NORM

Of course, we would do well to remember that for *Homo sapiens*, participating consciousness is the historical norm and the status quo. For more than 99 percent of human history, human beings have seen themselves as an integral part of the biosphere and the cosmos. Traditional cultures celebrated a merger with life. Human beings felt integrated with the natural world, a strand in the web, a branch on the tree of life. We were inside nature; our consciousness was participatory.

In the modern era, we have forced ourselves to become alienated observers of the universe. We have disconnected ourselves from our world in order to gain power and control. In the process, we have abandoned our bodies, our sensation and our flesh. This orientation, just as much as trans-fats, high-fructose corn syrup and video games, is the source of our modern physical malaise.

ADULTS ARE FROM MARS, CHILDREN ARE FROM EARTH

Our modern perspective is reflected in our approach to child rearing and our headlong push for accelerated development. For a few short years, we allow children to be Earthians with participatory consciousness. They can be impulsive, they can play, they can be subjective, passionate and emotional—at least until school age. But then, as soon as possible, we expect them to leave the Earth behind and become Martians. Suddenly, it's time to stop playing and start being objective. Give up emotion, give up the body and get down to the grim business of being dispassionate. Get your brain into the scientific-journalistic-academic-corporate-industrial complex of referenced documentation, annual reports, journal articles and disembodied professionalism. Whatever you do, get off the earth as soon as possible.

PUBLIC HEALTH

When it comes to matters of public health and epidemics of obesity, diabetes, heart disease and depression, many of us are turning to the Man from Mars for help. We expect that his objective, dispassionate viewpoint will help us make our bodies whole again. And so we produce an ever-expanding stream of research reports and studies, an avalanche of objective, dispassionate data on the breakdown of the modern human body. We hear it reported every day: another article in a journal of medicine, physiology or public health, written and edited by certified Martians, gives us one more redundant, data-centric account of our public health melt-down.

The problem is, it doesn't work. It can't work. How can we possibly use a disembodied perspective to diagnose and treat a disembodied public? How can getting out of your body be a solution to being out of your body? Our so-called "solution" is really just a reflection of the problem itself. Martian editors and administrators might give us an occasional kernel of interesting knowledge, but they will never give us the passion and participation we need to become truly healthy.

What we need are more Men from Earth and Women from Earth—people who participate with their bodies, emotion and passion. We need earth-bound primates who are expressive, artistic and impulsive, individuals who participate in the experience of being a mortal animal. We need people given to body-based action, even if it's not technically perfect or Martian-approved.

ONE FOOT ON EACH PLANET

As you can surely tell, I have grown tired of the Martians and their soulless data mongering. I am tired of footnotes, spreadsheets, references, journals and the dead voices of reason. I think it's obvious that our culture has gone too far in its Martian-worship.

But at the same time, I realize that there must be a yin-yang balance to this journey. That is, if we want to be completely functional and effective, we've got to be bilingual. We've got to do an apprenticeship on Mars and learn some basic Martian. It's essential to learn the scientific method, the power of objectivity and the virtues of distance. And then, once our apprenticeship is complete, let's give it the credit it deserves and get back to a truly creative life.

Sure, make a visit to Mars and take in the view. But please, whatever you do, don't get stuck there. It's a cold, hostile place that has nothing to offer our bodies. Earth is where this animal belongs. Take a trip to Mars for the education, but come back to Earth for your health.

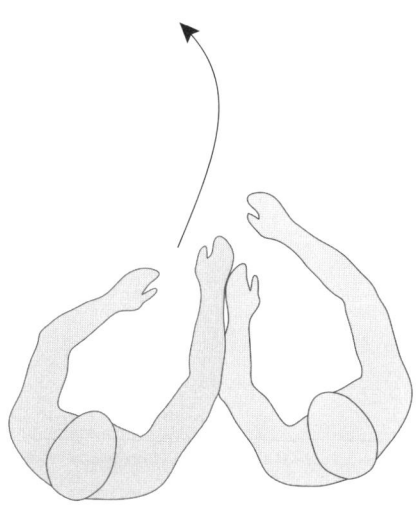

ANIMAL MAGNETISM:
STICKY WRIST, COACH LEADS WITH DIVERSE
MOVEMENT, ATHLETE FOLLOWS

Change Your Body, Change the World

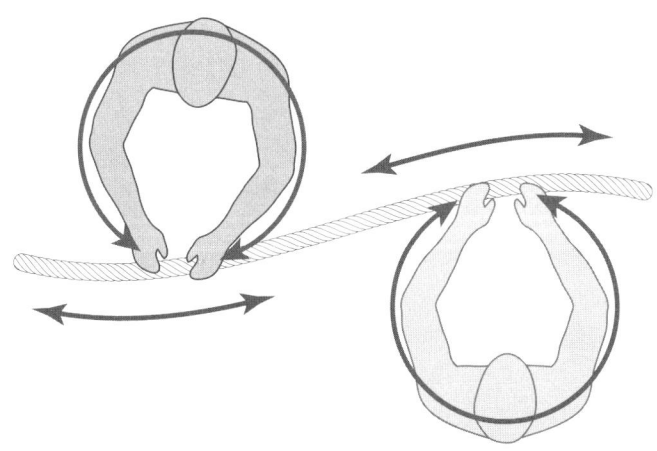

PARTNER-RESIST IN THE TRANSVERSE PLANE:
GIVE YOUR PARTNER SMOOTH RESISTANCE, USE YOUR CORE AND HIPS

WE INTERRUPT THIS BROADCAST

To the man who is afraid, everything rustles.

Sophocles

Is your mind tweaking your body? Are your thoughts and attitudes hampering your performance? Do your beliefs weaken your tissue, create fatigue or make you sick? Does your perception of the world impact your immune system, your cardiovascular system or your nervous system?

Maybe so. Probably so. Almost certainly so. Especially if you're a heavy consumer of modern media. Especially if you're addicted to stories of terror, greed, dysfunction, injustice, corruption and catastrophe.

Like it or not, it's all around us now. Just push the button and you can hear the rap any time of day or night: violence, hate, conflict, fear, anger, corruption, injustice, scandal...and on it goes, 24-7. Anxiety on tap—the modern news beat.

MIND SCULPTS THE BODY

As the discoveries of modern neuroscience are now making abundantly clear, the mind has a powerful effect on the body. The stories that we hear and tell are not neutral; they have profound impacts, not just on our thoughts, but on our flesh.

Chronic fear and stress, even if virtual, remote and abstract, can cause substantial damage to tissue throughout the body. Activate your sympathetic nervous system for weeks and months on end, and you'll wind up with thousands of dead neurons and millions of shrunken muscle fibers to show for it. Plus you'll become an irritable grouch, spreading your bile throughout the tribe.

It makes no difference, by the way, whether the anxiety rap comes from NPR, Air America or Fox. It doesn't matter if the grim prognosis comes from Adbusters, The Nation or American Heritage Foundation. It doesn't matter whether the hand-wringing comes from Michael Savage or Thom Hartman, Bill O'Reilly or Glenn Beck. It doesn't matter whether the name-calling comes from Ann Coulter or Randi Rhodes. Whatever the source, grim-speak wreaks havoc with our minds and in turn, our bodies. Our brains don't know the difference between right-wing bile or left-wing angst; it's all the same tone and has all the same effects. Bitterness and cynicism are stressful, no matter which side of the socio-political spectrum they happen to come from.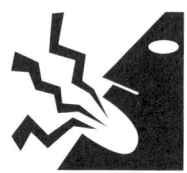

ADRENAL MEDIA

Unfortunately, we now live in a world in which fear, stress and anxiety are piped into our homes and automobiles in a near-constant stream. Modern media functions as a fear and anxiety amplifier, sharpening our perception of danger. Conflicts, real and imagined, become magnified. Discord is everywhere, systemic melt-down is imminent. Catastrophe looms, stalking our awareness like a hungry predator, threatening to pounce at any moment.

For marketing and advertising strategists, this is all as it should be of course. Their objective is simple after all: attract ears and eyeballs to the channel in question and keep them there. Contrast, conflict and catastrophe are ideal for this purpose. The human nervous system loves danger and destruction; the draw is almost irresistible. Show me a fight, some escalating tension and some drama, and my senses will perk up. Give me some terror, some fear and a looming catastrophe, and I'll reward you with my rapt attention.

By comparison, peace, health and happiness are dull; audience attention will drift and advertising money will go elsewhere. And so the programming decisions go in an entirely predictable direction: if it bleeds, terrifies or provokes, it leads. If a car explodes anywhere on the planet, it's newsworthy. If it pumps cortisol into the bloodstream, it goes above the fold or runs at the top of the hour. Stories of compassion, health, harmony and joy are left on the cutting room floor. In the world of fear media, happy, healthy people simply don't attract enough attention; for all practical purposes, they don't even exist.

OUR ALIEN ENVIRONMENT

This state of technological fear amplification is unprecedented in human history. In our Paleo world (life before media) there was plenty of stress to be had, but it was always local. A leopard might make a meal out of your best friend, a snake might sink his fangs into your leg or bad weather might chase your tribe across the grassland, but each of these challenges, however acute, tended to be temporary and was always in the moment.

Without modern media, there could be no awareness of remote emergencies or chronic catastrophes. Tribes on the other side of the world might be fighting epic battles against starvation, disease, tsunamis or one another, but you'd never know it. If all was well in your neighborhood, then all was well with your mind and body. Ignorance may not have been bliss, but it was almost certainly healthier.

In contrast, modern technology now allows us to feel anxious and upset over events that take place tens of thousands of miles away, well out of reach of normal sensation and awareness. It even allows us to feel anxious and upset over events that are only projected to occur. The problem is compounded by the fact that most of the ugly news that we're exposed to, whether true or hyped, usually describes events that we have almost no control over. Global warming, Afghanistan, Iraq, oil spills, the health care crisis: these problems are immense, far beyond the powers of most individuals to affect. And so, our relative sense of control actually begins to shrink. The brain senses a predicament, but we're unable to take action and our stress level rises.

STAYING INFORMED V. STAYING ALIVE

In the early days of our republic, most people believed that "staying informed" was an essential requirement for good citizenship. But what if staying informed also means exposing ourselves to a relentless stream of needless anxiety? What if staying informed means putting our health at risk? What if "staying informed" is actually a disguise for something else altogether—a distracting form of stimulation that serves some other psychological need?

A few years ago, Dr. Andrew Weil advocated an occasional "news fast" to help avoid the negative effects of overstimulation. And that was *before* 9/11, Iraq, Katrina, the oil spill and the daily flood of impossible problems that come into our brains at the top of every hour. It's beginning to look like Weil was ahead of his time. So, is it time to turn off the fear machines? I think it is.

This is not to suggest that ignorance and denial are the order of the day. It would be folly to disregard the problems of the modern world and give up our activism. But with an omnipresent, in-your-face information stream, there seems little danger that we might actually fall out of contact with world affairs.

Indeed, it would take an impressive effort of isolation to really get ourselves out of the loop. Instead, we need an approach that maintains both our health and our activism.

REQUIRED READING

Fortunately, there are alternative world views that counter-balance the fear-mongering. Rob Brezsny's *Pronoia is the Antidote for Paranoia* is an excellent example. Brezsny takes on "the purveyors of despair" and presents a life-affirming opposite: a celebration of wonder, exuberance and possibility. There's plenty of hippie-witchcraft and New Age playfulness in this book, but there are profound nuggets of serious wisdom as well, enough to derail even the most entrenched cynic. The spirit comes through loud and clear; happiness is in large measure a choice, a matter of attention.

We find a parallel track in Barbara Ehrenreich's book, *Dancing in the Streets*. Ehrenreich reminds us that celebrations, festivals and holidays have been a regular feature of normal human life for thousands of years. When our Europeans ancestors set sail to conquer the world, they were astonished to see a near-universal expression of enthusiasm among indigenous peoples. Everywhere they went, there was dancing, drumming and singing. Festivals were common; labor was modest. Joyful celebration seems to be the default for state for *Homo sapiens*. Happiness is the norm.

The Dalai Lama gives us much the same message in his recent books. Human nature, he tells us, is fundamentally gentle, compassionate and joyful. In *The Art of Happiness*, he reminds us of a truth that we are in imminent danger of forgetting; we are good animals and good people. Given a chance, we prefer to live in harmony with one another. It is only through repeated cycles of fear that we turn ugly and reactive. The Dalai Lama's message comes as a surprise to many of today's achieve-aholics, but there it is nonetheless: The purpose of life is to be happy.

BEAUTY, JOY, COMPASSION, HEALTH, APPRECIATION

So turn off the radio and tune out the fear. Stop pumping the cortisol channel. Forget about the imperialists, the corporatists, the dogmatists, the fascists, and the anarchists, at least for awhile. Instead, try being a joyful, intelligent activist—a joyist. Your body will thank you for it.

LIFEWAYS

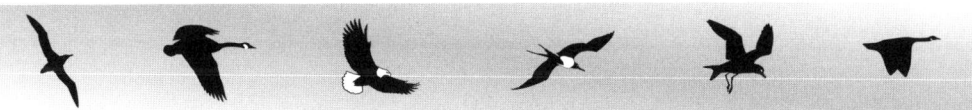

Change Your Body, Change the World

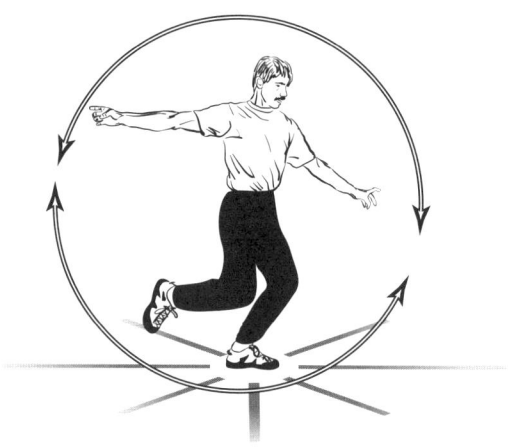

GIANT CIRCLES, ONE FOOT:
TRACE THE CIRCLE, BOTH DIRECTIONS, AS BIG AS YOU CAN

Change Your Body, Change the World

LET'S SEE...

Blessed are they who see beautiful things in humble places where other people see nothing.

Camille Pissarro

So here's a little test for you, a test of perception and vision. There's a line on one side of a whiteboard and it's about 12 inches long. You can see it clearly. On the other side of the whiteboard are three lines. One is obviously longer than the original, one is obviously shorter and one is obviously the same length.

I pose the question, "Which of the three lines matches up with the original?"

You hesitate for just a second, suspecting a trap, but there's really no doubt in your mind. You choose the correct line and get a gold star for your effort.

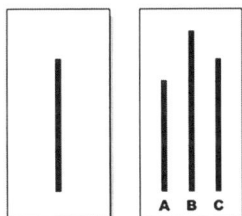

Now I run the test again, but this time I bring in a series of credible people (confederates) who consistently choose the "wrong" line. They declare with conviction that the longer line matches the original. One after another, they point to the long line and say "Yes, that's the match."

And now it's your turn. You try to cling to your original belief, but you're starting to waver. Doubt creeps into your mind and the longer line begins to look like a plausibly correct answer. Unconsciously, your perception begins to bend. When it's finally your turn, what will you say?

Well, it turns out that you might very well go with the group consensus. This is the finding of the famous Asch conformity experiments, led by social psychologist Solomon Asch in the 1950s. In a control group with no pressure to conform, only one subject out of 35 gave an incorrect answer. But when surrounded by individuals all voicing an incorrect answer, participants gave far more incorrect responses. This has become one of the most famous experiments in all of social psychology and has inspired similar research including Stanley Milgram's landmark work on obedience to authority.

TRIBAL INTELLIGENCE

When I first heard about this experiment and the fact that so many people would willingly revise and disown their personal perceptions, I was taken aback. "People are such lemmings," I mused, vowing that I would never fall victim to such a trap. I resolved that from that point forward, I would never go against the evidence of my own senses. I was no dupe; I would be a master of my own eyes and ears.

But years later, I revisited the Asch experiment from a new angle and suddenly the dupes didn't look so stupid after all. Now I was seeing things as an evolutionary biologist and wondering about the common human predicament, that is, life in a wild, natural and dangerous environment. I began to realize that this willingness to conform and adjust perception might actually be one of the most adaptive of all our behaviors, one that was key to our survival and development as a species.

To get the idea, you'll need to engage your imagination and put your mind squarely in habitat, deep in human prehistory. So step into the time machine, set the dial for 100,000 years ago and let 'er rip.

On arrival, you're going to notice a few things straight away. First, you're exposed. There are no walls to hide behind, no roofs to protect you from exposure, wind, scorching sun or rain. You might have a crude hut built from branches, grass and leaves, but this is only a thin layer of protection and an uncomfortable one at that. Basically, you're naked to everything the environment has to throw at you and danger is all around.

Human prehistory was thick with carnivores of all types: lions and leopards, as well as dangerous non-carnivorous creatures such as elephants, rhinos, hippos and enormous birds of prey. And even on good days when the carnivores were off hunting someone else, you'd still have a strong interest in finding food, which calls for exploration and learning your local bioregion.

But as a stand-alone human, you're at a considerable disadvantage. Your senses are sharp, but they just don't deliver as much information as you'd like. Your eyes are good, but only in the daytime and only when they're focused in front of you. Your ears aren't bad, but they could be better. Your sense of smell is weak, and depends on the wind. Your bare feet give you a good idea of texture, temperature and moisture, but you'd really like to know more. Taken together, your senses provide a fair but incomplete picture of your dangerous world.

So wouldn't it be great if you could somehow piggyback on other people's senses? Wouldn't you get a more complete view of your environment if you could harness the sensory capability of your tribe mates and hunting partners?

As it turns out, we are innately expert at doing precisely that. By virtue of our well-developed limbic brains and acute social awareness, we know how to share emotion and, to some degree, sensation with one another. By being sensitive to other people's experience, we effectively multiply our awareness of the world. Instead of one set of eyes, we now have many.

This is an enormous boon and gives us a huge survival advantage over solitary sensation. When hyper-social brains are linked, other people's experience becomes accessible to us; our knowledge of the world increases radically. Other people become sensory and knowledge multipliers. If you're good at reading other people's faces and bodies, you can learn quite a lot about your world. You can find more food and avoid becoming food yourself.

The same holds true for other animals in the wild by the way, especially grassland mammals such as antelope, kudu or zebra. Imagine that you're in your herd, grazing away. All is well, but you know instinctively that there's danger out there in the bush. You can't see as much as you'd like, but maybe your friends can see more, so you pay close attention. An ear twitches, a head rises a few degrees. Unconsciously, you register the smallest cues, piggybacking on the sensation of those around you. In this way, survival goes, not just to the fastest runner, but to those who are most alert to their neighbor's subtle sensory clues.

In the modern world, most of us have little conscious awareness of this contagion of sensory and emotional experience. Unless we actually go hunting in dangerous wild environments, we just don't feel the urgent drive to track one another's experience. Living in the lap of modern comfort and safety, we're not so motivated to watch one another's watching.

The closest thing to tribal sensory experience in the modern world is the small military force, the special ops unit on patrol in a hostile region. In this circumstance, danger is high and soldiers want as much information about the world as they can possibly get. This drives the unit towards sensory cohesion and social awareness. If the soldier next to you sees or hears something, you want to know about it immediately. You become hyper-alert to any clues in posture or facial expression. If your buddy's head turns sharply to the left, yours will likely follow. If his breathing changes, you'll take notice.

THE HYPER-SOCIAL CONTRACT

When primates "go social," the system begins to function like an external nervous system, or more precisely, an external sensory system. We may even go so far as to call it extra-somatic sensation or sensory contagion. I probe the world, not just with *my* eyes, ears, nose and skin, but also with *your* eyes, ears, nose and skin. And I do most of this unconsciously.

I call this capability for shared sensation and perceptual adjustment the "hyper-social contract." Implicitly and unconsciously we agree to modify our perceptions to fit prevailing patterns of group sensation and emotion. In other words, "I willingly give up some of my autonomy in exchange for more complete information about the world." It may sound crazy, but it's actually a pretty good deal.

This hyper-social contract has nothing to do with the abstract theories of civil organization advanced by philosophers such as Hobbes, Locke and Rousseau. Rather, it is basic to the human body and the human brain. Our mammalian limbic system is organized for social awareness: we are wired for affiliation, resonance and social attentiveness. All mammals share this capability, but human primates are the masters. We live with and through one another.

As much as Americans would like to celebrate the heroism of the intrepid individual, there can be no getting around the fact that our understanding of the world is a shared creation. Like it or not, we construct our knowledge of the world together. The process of shared perception and meaning is so powerful that it is almost inevitable; we can't not do it.

Stories, by the way, serve a similar purpose. We use story to share sensation, emotion and meaning. We use narrative to extend our knowledge of the world. Whether true or not, we absorb the total experience of the characters into our bodies and use it to interpret the world and help guide our actions.

In this sense, stories become part of the social nervous system.

So now, the Asch conformity experiment begins to take on a whole new meaning. People conform, not just because they're stupid or cowardly, (although they might well be) but because we're programmed to integrate other people's sensations, perceptions and judgments into our own experience. We pay attention to one other's attention and if there's a difference, we're willing to adjust our own. This isn't stupid. It's actually incredibly sophisticated.

THE MODERN CHALLENGE: GOOD NEWS, BAD NEWS

When sensory and emotional contagion operates in its natural context, it works great. A band of hyper-social hunters goes forth into unknown territory, in search of game and knowledge. They are alert for novelty and danger, each one sensitized not only to his own experience, but to the experience of others around him. Together, the band builds up a reliable image of terrain, plants, animals, opportunities and dangers around them. They avoid becoming prey and bring home some meat for the evening barbecue.

But the same capability, when applied in the modern world, can cause tremendous problems: mindless conformity, compulsive obedience to authority and in come cases, horrible atrocity. In other cases, it can lead to stress, isolation, hyperactivity, fragmented attention and learning disorders.

Back in the Paleolithic, sensory and emotional contagion worked best in small tribes and hunting parties in which emotion and sensation could be shared effectively to everyone's benefit. When everyone is sharing a similar predicament, there's a certain clarity, an ideal signal-to-noise ratio. All of your tribe mates have basically the same list of priorities: don't get eaten, find food and water, and learn the land.

But in the modern world, social living has become infinitely more complex. We're still hyper-social and unconsciously alert for other people's experience, but now millions of people are paying attention to all sorts of things, most of which have little or nothing to do with the natural world or a sustainable future. Instead, we are now besieged by "junk sensation" generated by our external nervous system.

What was once a finely tuned system for gathering information about the world has now become a vast and chaotic system that serves many different purposes. What was once highly focused (on survival in natural habitats) is now dispersed, displaced and radically diversified. Everyone, it seems, has a different set of priorities and consequently our attention is directed in thousands of different directions. And so, we seem to be left with only two choices: we can either allow ourselves to be swept up in socially-generated noise, or we can isolate, neither of which is ideal.

Social noise can create tremendous stress, especially for those who are tuned to other people's experience. Whereas tribal groups generated a coherent signal through shared predicament and experience, modern populations generate an immense amount of random, arbitrary and mostly useless emotional data that can deafen even the most stress-resistant among us. Our modern epidemic of stress-related disease, including depression, may be traceable, in part, to this hyper-noisy social-sensory system.

STRATEGIES FOR LIVING

So what are we to do with this sensory and emotional overload? If we are to be social at all, we must pay attention to one another, but this exposes us to the flood of distracting, random and arbitrary noise. What we can and must do is to learn ways to keep the noise at bay as we uncover the signal buried within. The recommendations are familiar to many, especially in the business world, but bear repeating.

First, clarify your vision. Unless you know exactly where you are going and what you're trying to do, noise will overwhelm your body, mind and mission. Now more than ever, it's essential to clearly identify personal and group objectives. What precisely are we trying to do in your predicament? What are you hunting? Without a goal, your emotions and sensations will become hijacked. Keep your eyes, ears and emotions focused on your target.

Second, be vigilant in protecting your attention. Practice triage and build firewalls. Lay down strict personal guidelines regarding who and what you pay attention to. Don't allow your awareness to be compromised by noisy trivia. Practice saying no to distractions. Focus on content and look for solid reference points.

Unfortunately, these guidelines often feel artificial and even unnatural. Such strategies were completely unnecessary in the Paleolithic and many of us find such discipline difficult and troubling. Given the chance, we tend to slide back into our primal habits of attention and make ourselves vulnerable to the modern noise machine. Nevertheless, disciplined attention has become a necessity in the modern world. If we slacken our efforts too much, we'll get buried.

PAY ATTENTION TO ATTENTION

Finally, we must take to heart a lesson that's becoming increasingly obvious as social neuroscience uncovers ever more connectivity between people. Because we are so given to sharing sensation, emotion and meaning as we build up our understanding of the world, it now becomes clear that *what we look at matters*.

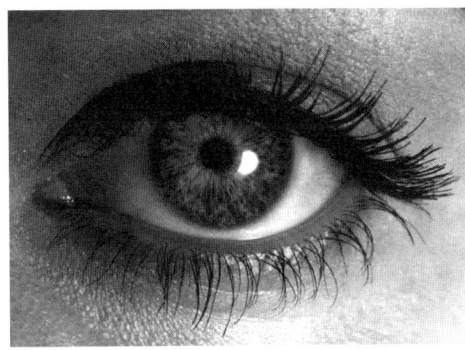

In other words, there's an ethical responsibility that comes with social attention and shared sensation. We are responsible, in some measure, for the emotional state of each another. We are also responsible, to some degree, for the sensory and perceptual experience of one another. Our search for meaning ultimately affects other people's lives.

When we understand that every act of attention and imagination is potentially contagious, we suddenly realize that it makes a difference whether we attend to substance or junk. It makes a difference whether we attend to darkness or to light, to conflict or to peace. Attention, in other words, is not neutral.

With so much talk of junk food in our conversations about health, we also need to consider the negative effects of junk attention, junk sensation and junk emotion. Focusing our minds on cheap, worthless or negative qualities of the world is likely to be just as dangerous as gorging on high-fructose corn syrup and trans-fats.

The process works in the positive direction as well of course. That is, it makes a difference when we direct attention towards things that are beautiful, natural, courageous, promising or positive. It makes a difference when we look at habitat and bioregional qualities. It makes a difference when we choose to appreciate art, music, science and learning. It makes a difference when we stop dwelling on the negative and focus on the creative bounty of nature and the human imagination.

Our experience, however intimate and personal, ultimately gets shared. Not explicitly perhaps, but unconsciously, through non-verbal cues and powerful social contagions.

The implications are clear: look for truth and beauty, peace and integrity. Look towards strength and compassion. Look for light. Use your sensation and experience as a contribution to the tribe. Create meaning that's worth sharing.

You may not save your tribe from the carnivores of the grassland, but you might help us navigate our way to a sustainable and meaningful future.

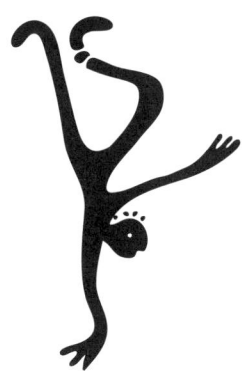

LIFE ON THE MISSISSIPPI

There comes a time in every rightly-constructed boy's life when he has a raging desire to go somewhere and dig for hidden treasure.

Mark Twain
The Adventures of Tom Sawyer

So here we are, stuck in the middle of an epic and paradoxical predicament. The modern world has its share of worthy pleasures, but it also generates a colossal flood of junk and confusion. Our minds are swamped a sea of swirling abstractions, competing claims and exploding information. Science tells us a great deal about the nature of reality, but offers little guidance in the art of living.

Like many, I have gone in search for grounded truth in the art of living and have sought my own models of common sense. As an avid reader of Mark Twain, my natural choice is Tom Sawyer and Huck Finn, the boys described in Samuel Clemens' classics, *The Adventures of Tom Sawyer* and *The Adventures of Huckleberry Finn*. These boys lived in Hannibal, Missouri, in the middle of the 19th century. Their lives were rural and simple, yet incredibly adventurous. Their daily experience was highly physical, engaging and robust.

There are many reasons to like Tom and Huck as grounding personalities in the world of health. First, they lived in a time before modernity really hit the fan. Their family livelihoods were based on agriculture of course, but there was plenty of hunting, fishing, playing and above all, walking. No cars, no computers, no concrete, no couches, no air-conditioners. There was copious contact with nature and a generous sense of temporal affluence. That is, people actually had time to live.

Tom and Huck engaged their world directly with their bodies and their lives were untainted by adult intervention in matters of physical fitness and health. They were basically wild animals, playing their way to physical development and health. They received instruction in basic literacy and conduct, but that was about it. In essence, Tom and Huck were both autodidacts; in terms of physical education, they were almost entirely self-taught. Their inquiries into life were curiosity-driven, practical and relevant.

THE TOM AND HUCK LIFESTYLE

For those of us who are mired in the trappings of modernity, it's essential that we revisit the era of Tom and Huck and get a sense of what their young lives were like. It was only a few generations ago, but the experience seems light years from the way we live today. For Tom and Huck, a typical summer night might go like this: Stay awake in bed until after dark and wait for the "owl hoot" that means your fellow adventurer has arrived outside. Climb out the window and slide down the drain pipe, jump onto the shed roof and climb to the ground. Walk a few miles to a hill outside of town, carrying shovels or a dead cat to ward off warts. Wait until the light of the moon casts a long shadow in just the right spot and then start digging for buried treasure. Dig deep into the ground, sweating hard until you hit rock, then try somewhere else. Later, you might visit a graveyard or a "haunted house," then run like the wind from the bad guys.

During a summer day, you might walk down to the river, "borrow" a boat, row out to Jackson Island and spend the rest of the day swimming and climbing trees. Or, you might explore the local cave and even get lost for a few days. You might flee down the Mississippi on a raft, pitting your body against the elements. Along the way, you might pull into shore, walk long distances between towns or steal some chickens that "weren't resting too comfortable." Every day was physical.

Tom and Huck lived a life that we now understand as inherently healthy. Not only did they walk long distances on most days, they also understood the folly of footwear and avoided it whenever possible. Shoes were for Sunday, a painful and unpleasant departure from normal living. By avoiding footwear, they kept their feet, ankles, knees and hips smart and fast. Tom and Huck didn't look like athletes, but their bodies were highly intelligent and fully capable of navigating their world.

Nutrition was never a problem because there really wasn't much to eat and all of it was organic, locally grown food. Meat was good, but so were the vegetables; these kids were hungry because they were in constant motion. No drive-thru, chemically-enhanced speed eating: do your chores and later, you'll get to eat.

Above all, Tom and Huck lived a play-based, adventure-based lifestyle. Their fantasy lives were rich and they made do with the simplest of toys. There were chores to be done and fences to be whitewashed, but they did their best to avoid it. The mere sight of a steamboat churning up the river could spark an entire afternoon of mimicking and role-playing, entirely without the direction of adults or electronic devices.

As for physical experience, we can be sure that Tom and Huck never did a work-out or set foot in a gym. They never practiced organized sports. They never counted sets or reps. They never wore heart-rate monitors or pedometers. They never logged their progress on spreadsheets.

And yet, it's safe to assume that the Toms and Hucks of the 19th century were healthy and physically educated. Sure, there were injuries and the occasional threat of infectious disease, but there was very little of the obesity, diabetes and physical apathy that afflicts us today. Tom and Huck were not super-athletes, but they were super-healthy and highly adaptable, ready to take on a wide variety of physical challenges, from cave exploration to long-distance river travel. Tom and Huck's success in navigating their world is proof enough: these kids were physically educated and exceptionally clever.

WHAT WOULD TOM AND HUCK DO?

So what would Tom and Huck have to say about our modern crisis of the human body? What would they say about the plight of the modern American and our frantic, hyper-stressed, aphysical culture?

They would be flummoxed no doubt, shocked to see how incredibly disempowered we have become: a vast population of weak and helpless individuals, increasingly dependent on technology for the most basic functions of life. A world of work-addicted people, with never enough time to sit on the porch or explore the world on foot. A nation of people so completely dependent on automobiles that many can scarcely walk, their sensory-motor circuits having gone dormant from lack of use.

Tom and Huck would be mystified and resolve to have none of it. They would build a raft and head down river, hiding out during the day and floating nights. They would set out the lines and catch some fish, liberate a few chickens and try to steer clear of the big towns. Along the way, they'd have more adventures. They'd get hot and cold, hungry and tired. They'd flee from thunderstorms in the afternoon, see the stars at night and marvel at the wonders of the natural world.

BE LIKE TOM, BE LIKE HUCK

The human body is in crisis, there can be no question. As adults, we propose all sorts of adultified solutions: more and better technology, more and better administration, more programs, more of everything that got us into this predicament in the first place. But from Tom and Huck's vantage point, we are missing the target by a thousand miles. We are missing the fundamentals of simple physical living and play-based adventure. We desperately need Tom and Huck to get us back on course.

Conventional wisdom holds that "it takes a village to raise a child." But in our case, we might do better to say "it takes a child to raise a village." Or, more specifically, it takes two sensible boys to show us the folly of our ways.

So forget the policy recommendations cranked out by the big institutions. Forget the expensive, energy-sucking devices that promise the ultimate in physical conditioning. And while you're at it, forget the technicolor role models. Forget Tiger. Forget Lance. Forget Laird. Forget every big-money athlete, every gold-plated champion and every Photoshopped poser that lives on a magazine cover. Get some authentic physical experience in the natural world.

Be like Huck.

Be like Tom.

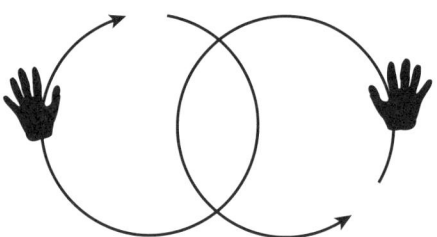

WAX ON, WAX OFF:
ALL SIZES, ALL PLANES, ALL STANCES

LEARNING FROM THE INSIDE OUT

More words count less.

Lao Tzu
Tao te Ching

Physical education is about learning, we can all agree on that. But what's your style? How do you learn new things? Well, that probably depends on your genes, your personal history and your preferences. It also depends on your culture.

Consider my experience as a beginning drum student. My teacher's name is Ibrahima and he's the real thing, a master African drummer. He played with Stevie Wonder for awhile and was once the head choreographer for the National Ballet of Senegal. Not only is he a master drummer, he's a dancer and singer as well. He's physically educated, happy and healthy.

Once a week we gather for our drum class, the Americans seated with Ibrahima in a circle. Ibrahima greets us and lays down a pattern of tones, bass notes and slaps. He expects us to play back his "call" but instead, before the vibrations even settle out of the air, we reach for our notebooks. Almost in unison, every last one of us grabs for paper and pen, desperate to capture the pattern before it fades from memory.

Ibrahima watches this spectacle and breaks out into hysterical laughter. "What are you doing?" he asks in his French-Senegalese accent. Someone offers an explanation, but it goes nowhere fast. We tell him that we need to capture the song so that we can remember it, but he rejects our reasoning outright. "Stop writing," he instructs bluntly. "That's not going to help you. Learn it with your body. Learn it with your muscles. Learn it with your flesh. Trust your body. That's how you learn it." He shakes his head, astonished at the magnitude of our ignorance.

Embarrassed, we reluctantly put down our notebooks, although some of us continue to scribble furiously, ink on palms and forearms, desperate to secure the fleeting rhythm into print. Ibrahima laughs again and lays down the riff once more, demanding that we play it whether we're ready or not. "Start playing," he instructs. "You can figure it out once you're in motion."

OUTSIDE-IN V. INSIDE-OUT

Obviously, we Westerners are out of our element here. Raised to be note-takers and abstractionists, we feel compelled to write everything down. We don't trust our bodies or our memory. And so, we try to capture the music in symbols, hoping that we can sort it out later.

What we're attempting to do, of course, is to use our conscious, cognitive brains to instruct our tissue. Our method is top-down: Learn by abstraction and then direct the body from above. Explain it first, then execute the act; we believe in a system of command-and-control. Or, to put it another way, we try to learn from the outside-in.

Ibrahima on the other hand, believes in learning from the inside out. Start with the action and explain it later, if you must. Learn by doing. Learn it first with your tissue, your flesh. Muscle has tremendous memory for movement, so why not start there? Get some motion going so you'll have something to work with. This is how drum and dance has been taught in Africa for generations. No instruction manuals, no abstract theories, just gobs of immersion and authentic experience.

Ibrahima may not be aware of it, but his philosophy is backed up by recent discoveries in neuroscience. We now know that learning is best accomplished by physical action and engagement, in other words, by doing. There is simply no better way. Sensory and motor circuits adapt to how they are used, not by some conceptual model imposed from above. We learn movement by moving; everything else is a side-show.

THE BODY IS A MUSICAL INSTRUMENT

Musicians everywhere are united on this score. Theoretical abstractions don't carry much weight in music education; it's time-on-task that makes the difference. Learn to play by playing. Learn to move by moving. Keep at it. Immerse yourself in the process and participate fully. Practice, practice, practice. Abstract knowledge is nice if you can get it, but it's action that makes the musician.

In this sense, music and athletics are simply different expressions of the same physical education process. Africans have known this for a long time, but in the West we have yet to realize the common ground between music and movement. We segregate athletics and music into different departments, often located at opposite ends of campus. We use different curriculums and require that athletic and music teachers undertake entirely different courses of study and earn separate credentials.

But this isolation and segregation reveals a deep misunderstanding of physical learning. In fact, the musician and the athlete are engaged in a learning process that is far more similar than it is different. Ultimately, the biggest difference between the musician and the athlete is that the athlete works with big muscles of the butt, thighs and core, while the musician works with smaller muscles of the fingers, arms or mouth. But both artists are ultimately after the same objective: quality movement that's smooth, powerful and lively. Both are working the nervous system, sensation and motor feedback loops to produce highly coordinated, orchestrated movement.

In fact, as a thought experiment, let's try putting music teachers in charge of physical education physical educators in charge of music. Yes, there would be a transition period with plenty of noise and wasted effort in the process, but ultimately everything would work out very nicely indeed. Musicians and coaches are both physical performance teachers after all.

So let's get back to the fundamentals. Leave the abstractions for another day. Get some movement going, then refine it as you go. Play the music, play the body, play the drum. It's all the same thing.

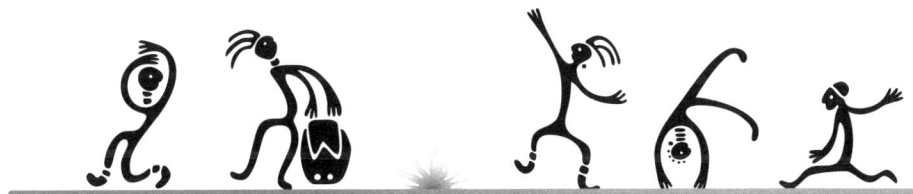

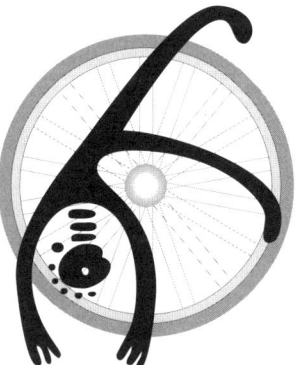

PLAYSTATE

> I played with an idea, and grew willful; tossed it into the air; transformed it; let it escape and recaptured it; made it iridescent with fancy, and winged it with paradox.
>
> Oscar Wilde

> This is the real secret of life—to be completely engaged with what you are doing in the here and now. And instead of calling it work, realize it is play.
>
> Alan Watts

Are you ready to play?
Right now, this instant?
Are you ready to mix things up and embrace new sensations, movements and ideas?

Are you leaping from one challenge to the next, rearranging the elements of your world in new and exciting combinations? Or are you grinding away on whatever's in front of you, wishing it would just go away?

It all comes down to a simple question: Are you in a playful state of mind and body? If so, what led you to be here? If not, why not? And how can you get back in?

SERIOUS BUSINESS

Welcome to the paradox of play. On first glance, play might appear to be a trivial practice of childhood that's suitable for kindergarten and not much else. But as we look deeper into animal behavior, education and performance, we come to the surprising conclusion that play is actually a matter of supreme importance. Play is pivotal to success in virtually every field of human endeavor, from athletics and art to business and relationships. And it is vital to the health of body, mind and spirit.

Like language, music and dance, play is a human universal. It is common to every culture and is widespread in the animal world, especially in animals of higher intelligence. Play facilitates learning, development and functional behavior. In fact, play occurs at precisely the same time in the lifespan when neural growth is at its peak.

Our most successful artists, athletes and creators are those who remember how to play. They know how to create conditions for nurturing the play instinct and how to get back in when they fall out of play. If we can learn to recognize this state and the elements that lead us in and out, we just might be able to enter it at will and stay there a little bit longer.

Unfortunately, many of us suffer from a kind of play amnesia as we grow older; we not only forget the actual events of our youth but even more tragically, we forget the feeling that led us to play in the first place. Consumed by work and continuously pressed for time, we triage play out of our lives and find ourselves stressed, depressed and anxious.

As children, our play instinct was an almost unstoppable force, a central organizing theme for our existence. The whole point of being alive was to play; everything else was a mere distraction, an interruption between play bouts. Instinctively, we knew that play was vital to survival, physicality and success. The drive to play eclipsed nearly every other consideration; we played to live and lived to play.

But as we entered adulthood, we began to spend less time in the play state. Adults pushed us towards practicality, planning and delayed gratification. Over time, we began to take on this role for ourselves; the force of discipline and play-inhibition began to come from within our own brains, specifically from the prefrontal cortex.

This fascinating chunk of brain tissue has several functions including impulse control and inhibition of the emotionally rich limbic system. In the young human animal, development of the prefrontal cortex lags behind the rest of the brain and doesn't fully mature until the early 20s. That's why young people tend to be more emotionally expressive and creative; it's also why they tend to be more irresponsible. When the prefrontal cortex finally comes on line, young adults become more adept at dampening emotional states including fear, anger, sadness and of course, creative play.

This is a good news, bad news situation. On one hand, a mature prefrontal cortex gives us the emotional control to function in a complex social world and to delay gratification. We find that, by inhibiting our emotional lives, we can accomplish great things. We can get jobs, write books, earn advanced degrees and plan for the future. In fact, society rewards us handsomely for our acts of emotional inhibition. We are paid well for the ability to sit still for long periods, work deeply with detail and delay our personal needs.

Herein lies the trap: we find that inhibition pays off and we begin to practice it habitually. Even when not required to do so, we continue to exercise prefrontal authority over limbic emotion. And in the process, we lose touch with our creativity and our sense of play. In extreme cases, play disappears entirely from our lives and we become dull, joyless drones.

So, we need remedial education. We need to remember what play feels like. And most importantly, we need strategies for getting back in when we fall out.

REMEMBERING THE PLAY STATE

So let's refresh our memory. Maybe it's been awhile and you can't quite remember what the play state feels like. Try to imagine your last genuinely playful experience. You may have to go back years, even decades, but do it. Close your eyes. Think about the entire experience: the environment, the social setting, the time of day, your clothing, the way your body felt, your sense of time and self.

It's different for everyone, of course, but there seem to be some common elements that hold true. When we're in the play state, we're

- relaxed but energized
- curious, experimental, creative
- engaged, focused, absorbed
- present-oriented, outside of time
- lacking in self-awareness
- interested in the experience for its own sake
- awash in the sense of possibility, options, opportunity

FLOW

The play state shares a good many characteristics with "flow." As described by Mihaly Csikszentmihalyi in his landmark book *Flow: The Psychology of*

Optimal Experience, flow is the mental state in which a person is fully immersed in what he or she is doing. Csikszentmihalyi's description sounds very similar to our play state. His list includes:

- concentrating and focusing
- a loss of the feeling of self-consciousness, the merging of action and awareness
- distorted sense of time
- balance between ability level and challenge
- a sense of personal control over the situation or activity.
- a sense that the activity is intrinsically rewarding, so there is an effortlessness of action.
- a sense of absorption; the focus of awareness is narrowed to the activity itself.

The parallels between flow and the play state are striking and the two states seem almost interchangeable. If you're really playing, you're in flow. If you're in flow, you're either playing or working in deep concentration. Either way, you're in a state that not only feels good, it 's immensely healthy, practical and ultimately productive.

What we're seeing here is an ideal state for living. When we're in flow or play, mind-body integration is at its highest. If we looked close enough, we'd see a balance in the autonomic nervous system of the flow-state player. We'd see optimal levels of activity in the sympathetic and parasympathetic nervous systems. We'd be energized, but relaxed; alert but calm. Stress hormones would be circulating at low levels, enough to stimulate attention and promote learning, but not so much as to trigger anxiety or tissue damage.

SKILL DEVELOPMENT

When we think about the ebb and flow of the play state and our desire to enter into it, we begin to realize that there's a genuine aptitude here. Finding the sweet spot of play is not a matter of random groping. Rather, there's a skill and a method. With practice, we can learn to recognize the play state and position ourselves to take advantage of play-friendly forces and influences. This also implies the ability to coax ourselves back into play. It suggests a sense of resilience and the ability to rebound after hardship, distraction or calamity.

So let's suppose you've fallen out of the play state. You're tired, bored, depressed or uninspired and now you'd like to get some bounce in your body, mind and spirit. The process begins by creating the right context. Like health itself, play will return when conditions are favorable. So, while we can't force the issue with a strict program of cause and effect, there are some things that we can do to improve the odds:

START WITH THE BODY

Start with the body and look for autonomic balance. If you're too stressed, you're in fight-flight-freeze and you're not going to be playing much. Learn the tricks for lowering your stress: breathing, vigorous movement, reframing, social support. Physical play is promising here because it creates a virtuous circle: play reduces stress which in turn allows creative play to emerge more completely.

NEW MOVES

As you move your body, stay alert for new postures, positions, movements and sensations. Let your body send fresh feedback to your brain. Try a new physical discipline or a fresh approach to an old favorite. Don't be afraid to look foolish: strange new movements are the foundation of creative physicality and athleticism.

BALANCE CHALLENGE AND SKILL

Look for a playful flow state by adjusting the difficulty of the challenge. Things that are too easy or too hard discourage both flow and play. Step back from your predicament and tweak the challenge so that you're in the sweet spot of perfect difficulty. Be more ambitious or less so.

TURN THINGS UPSIDE DOWN AND BACKWARDS

Set up a creative rhythm; make a mess, clean it up, then repeat. Get into the mess-making; let order break down. Embrace entropy, let things fall apart into new combinations and arrangements. Give up on order and perfect safety. Leave some things to chance; embrace risk and ambiguity. Play is often dangerous. You can clean it all up later.

GO NEO

Expose yourself to something completely different. Travel, both globally and locally, both physically and mentally. Put yourself into a fresh predicament. Play a different role; write yourself a new job title and a new story. Feed on novelty.

CREATE AN ENRICHED ENVIRONMENT

Customize your play space for maximum creative conditions. Tweak the layout, the order and the relationships. More light, more color, more novelty, more inspiration and more change.

DREAM IMPOSSIBLE THINGS BEFORE BREAKFAST

Practice outrageous and courageous brainstorming, completely without concern for practicality. Ignore the critic. The editor, whether internal or external, should come late to the game, if at all. Give him the day off or better yet, an extended vacation.

OXYMORONS

Nourish some oxymorons by combining normally contradictory elements. *Oxymoron* is from Greek oxy ("sharp" or "pointed") and moros ("dull"). Polarities are powerful stimulants to play and learning. As Tom Ward, editor, *Journal of Creative Behavior* put it, "To enhance creativity, merge two previously separate concepts that are in conflict with one another. For example, combinations such as 'friendly enemy' and 'healthful illness.' The more discrepant the concepts, the more likely they are to result in novel properties."

CHASE DOWN A FASCINATION, NURTURE A HOLY CURIOSITY

What are you most curious about in this world? What do you really want to know more about? If you had unlimited resources, what would you investigate? What discipline would you study? What skill would you develop?

FIND PLAYFUL ROLE MODELS

Start spending more time with playful people. Make a list of the most playful people in your life and call them up. If you're stuck, imagine what a playful person would do in your predicament. Think of the most playful person you know; what would he or she do in your situation?

CHANGE THE BOUNDARIES

An overly expansive range of possibility can stagger the imagination and bring us to a standstill. On the other hand, if the range of options is too narrow, it can stifle our sense of movement. Try moving the fences in either direction.

TIMELESS

Think outside the clock. Think back to childhood and your life before time consciousness. Did you ever care how long a thing took? Did you ever give the slightest thought to duration? It was the adventure that mattered.

ABANDON SELF

Ignore the self and get into process. Get into the act of learning, training and experiencing. Focus on the material, the curiosity, the object of your imagination.

PERMISSION TO FAIL

To get back into play, we've got to give ourselves license to make errors and to produce lousy work, lots of it. Creativity is inherently wasteful. Nature's exuberance generates millions of forms that die, all so that a select few can thrive. All artists generate a lot of material, most of which gets set aside or thrown away. No matter; it's the generation that matters.

MASTERY

So what's the potential here? How far can we go with our playskills? The short answer is that we don't know because, as a culture, we haven't really tried. In fact, we spend untold millions of hours doing our level best to squelch the play impulse at every turn. We tell ourselves that play is a threat to productivity, and in the short term it probably is. But when we stretch our time horizon out just a little, from the urgent to the important, we begin to see that play is not just fun, it's powerful, transformative and essential to growth and sustainability.

So perhaps it's time to consult the imagination. Let's imagine a strange and mysterious culture in a land far, far away, a powerful race of men and women that valued play and actively trained for resilience and exuberance.

These play masters were adept at turning adversity into play. Their play awareness was honed to extreme sensitivity. They could recognize the precise instant when their minds and bodies began to fall out of play. And once outside, they knew how to rebound and let themselves back in.

The stories would have been legendary. In practice, these play shamans could turn fear into play. They could turn anger into play. They could take any negative experience—depression, illness, stress, loss—and turn it into something that moved, something of interest, something with promise. In reality, the play masters were just as weak, vulnerable and confused as any of us, but they had the knowledge, the skill and the training to make the difference. It was all the same challenge to them; take the adversity and transform it into something that moves.

And have fun doing it.

Why would we do it any other way?

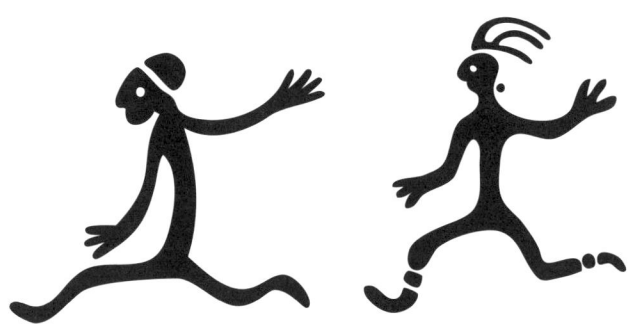

WELCOME TO THE NEO-PALEO

> The friendly and flowing savage, who is he? Is he waiting for civilization, or is he past it, and mastering it?
>
> Walt Whitman

When the going gets tough, many of us long for a simpler time. Squeezed by stress and punished by our modern predicament, our imagination drifts off to some golden age, a time when the pressures of life weren't quite so onerous, or were at least more comprehensible. Some of us long for childhood, while others dream of the lifestyle of our old home towns. In whatever form, we long for an escape to utopia.

Without question, the modern world *is* tough. The sedentary living, the relentless pressure to produce, the disorienting effects of modern technology; our bodies, minds and spirits feel disconnected and adrift. Not only do we feel out of place, we feel a disturbing trend of increasing alienation from life-giving habitats and behavior. The more we learn about the body-hostile qualities of our modern environment, the more we look for escape into a more natural and comforting realm.

For some of us, that realm has become the Paleolithic. The *paleo*, many of us have come to believe, was a time of physical purity and boundless health, a time of harmony with land, tribe and the cosmos as a whole. As the insanity of the modern world closes in on us, we look back, way back, for a sense of refuge and relief.

The word *paleo* simply means "old," "ancient" or "prehistoric." The *Paleolithic era* refers to "the old stone age," the period of human prehistory distinguished by the development of the first stone tools. It extends from the introduction of stone tools by hominids such as *Homo habilis* 2.5 million years ago to the introduction of agriculture around 10,000 years ago.

Today, many of us simply use the word Paleo as shorthand for "before modernity hit the fan." And now, as human evolution becomes more widely recognized as the true source of our physical identity, we're seeing a proliferation of Paleo programs and philosophies around the world. We now have Paleo diets, cookbooks, recipes, fitness programs, books and blogs. Paleo is getting big and is bound to get bigger in the years to come.

ON ONE HAND...

So what are we to make of this modern dream of an ancient past? On the one hand, our interest in all things Paleo is exciting and refreshing. It suggests that people are looking deeper for a sense of meaning and identity. We're finally breaking free from the synthetic, stifling atmosphere of big box gyms and going in search of our authentic physical roots.

It's also clear that there's valid medical reasons for this renewed interest in our deep past. The "Paleo lifestyle," as we understand it today, looks to be perfectly congruent with the form and function of the human body. All available evidence points to the health-positive effects of living on the land, eating real food, following circadian rhythms and living in tribes. A flood of new research confirms this belief.

ON THE OTHER...

It's tempting to dive right into the Paleo philosophy and lifestyle, but reflection is in order. The main challenge is our considerable ignorance. Despite a flood of recent discoveries in paleontology, molecular biology and evolutionary biology, we really don't know that much about the Paleolithic or the lifestyle of our ancestors. In short, much of our current Paleo-mania is based on fragmentary information and pure out-and-out romance.

For many, the image of the Paleo lifestyle is little more than a cartoon snapshot of an immensely deep, rich and complex period of history. We read a few books, watch a couple of documentaries and we've got the picture: the intrepid hunter-gatherer, club in hand, body wrapped in fur, running an ultra-marathon across the grassland, chasing down the evening meal.

Once we've got this snapshot in mind, we expand it into a complete world view. The mind grabs hold and starts filling in detail with conjecture and assumptions. We begin to fall in love with the image we've created and go on to build entire philosophies, lifestyles, businesses and cults.

In fact, we really don't know that much about Paleo peoples or their lifestyles. Yes, we know that our ancestors lived in wild, natural habitats and that they probably made their living with some combination of hunting, scavenging and gathering. It's safe to assume that they lived in tribes and that they moved around a good deal, probably walking long distances on most days, usually barefoot.

This portrait of human prehistory is probably accurate, but it remains a caricature of what must have been a tremendously rich and varied story. What gets lost in our over-simplified narrative is the vast diversity of land, climate, plants, animals and people.

The Paleolithic was not a static monolith of natural history. During this period of over 2 million years, there were wild fluctuations in every dimension of habitat and human experience. To get a sense of this diversity, all that's necessary is to study the terrain, landscapes and habitats of modern day Africa. Even a short airplane flight reveals an astonishing range of landforms, sometimes radical differences within a single square mile. Deserts, grasslands, wetlands and forests lie in surprising proximity to one another. In all likelihood, conditions were similar in the Paleolithic.

Change was constant throughout this period. Tectonic plates crashed into one another, buckling the land and building mountains. Massive volcanoes erupted periodically, spewing forth billions of tons of ash, blanketing the Serengeti and other landscapes. Climactic change was continuous: drying and cooling led to a thinning of the forest of East Africa. Droughts and extended monsoons came and went, drenching and dehydrating entire landscapes.

In addition to climate and habitat diversity, there was clearly a diversity of hominids—pre-human bipedal primates. Paleontologists have clearly identified at least a dozen or more, ranging from *Australopithecus* to *Homo habilis*, *Homo ergaster* and *Homo erectus*. Like all animals, these hominids must have inhabited different ecological niches, eaten different foods and migrated in different patterns. It's certain that there would have been huge variations in lifestyle.

Homo sapiens appeared on the scene about 200,000 years ago, but we can be sure that diversity was still the name of the game. Organized into small tribes, these tribes developed unique strategies, methods and cultures for survival. Each tribe had its own relationship to habitat and its own patterns of hunting, gathering and migration.

This would have meant profound differences in lifestyle from region to region. Some tribes practiced highly active persistence hunting, while others were more inclined to wait and let the game come to them. Some would have gathered more than others. Some would have fished and gathered in aquatic habitats. Given this diversity of habitat and peoples, it is folly to say that there was or is a single Paleo lifestyle.

FOOD

Our cartoon version of the Paleo becomes obvious as soon as we start talking about something called "the Paleo diet." Experts attempt to make a case that our primal ancestors ate in some consistent, regular pattern that is optimal for modern humans living today.

But this simply cannot be the case. Primal peoples must have eaten all sorts of things. They were hungry opportunists and their habitat was always in flux. We can be certain that there were large regional and seasonal variations. Were we meat-eaters or were we more inclined towards a vegetarian diet? We'll never really know the full story. We can study modern-day tribes such as the Hadza in Tanzania or the !Kung in Botswana, but these are just two examples out of hundreds of possibilities.

We do know that cooking made a tremendous difference in human evolution, a point driven home by Richard Wrangham in *Catching Fire: How Cooking Made us Human.* But this complicates the issue even further: the ability to cook also gave us the ability to consume a far wider variety of foods than every before, making it even less likely that we can point to a single Paleo foodstyle.

TRUE PALEO

We'll never really know all we'd like about human prehistory, but what about Paleo in today's world? Aren't some native peoples living authentic Paleo right now?

Almost certainly not. Without exception, native peoples have been severely impacted by colonialism and modernity. Entire cultures have been destroyed, but even more importantly, the connection between native peoples and the land has been almost completely severed. Tribes have been relocated from one region to another or to reservations. Land has been fenced or partitioned off for cattle, mining or wildlife reserves.

Consequently, most native people are now adopting modern ways or living in desperation, trying to get enough to eat in lands that are no longer familiar to them. Even in cases where primal peoples live in their original habitats, they have adopted new ways of living. Native peoples in the Arctic now use snowmobiles and rifles to hunt. Bushmen in Africa use metal arrow points and knives.

There may be some lingering pockets of authentic Paleo-style living in New Guinea, the Amazon rainforest or the outback of Australia, but there seems little hope that this lifestyle will persist for much longer. Like it or not, true Paleo no longer exists.

A HARD LIFE

It's easy to romanticize the Paleo, but when we really consider the reality of it, we find a fresh appreciation for the pleasures *and* the pain. Yes, we can long for the immensity and the intensity of raw physical living. The Paleo would have given us Nature in all her glory: spectacular beauty, naked sensation and total immersion in the here and now. Our bodies and our spirits would have thrived under these conditions.

But the Paleo, whatever it may have been, was not all comfortable health and spiritual delight. For all the psychic and physical appeal, the hardships would have been enormous: sleeping on the ground or in trees, suffering heat, cold, drought and an uncertain food supply. The people of the Paleolithic, like most wild animals, lived in intimate proximity to dirt and death.

People of the Paleo were often hungry, hot or cold, scraped up, bruised and dirty, often besieged by insects. No toothpaste or hot showers. No antiseptics, bandages or pain meds. Daily life was rugged. And as for sex, that would have probably have been brief, intense and reproductive. Without a soft bed, candles and music, what more could you hope for?

GET SERIOUS

But let's suppose you've considered both the ups and downs of "going Paleo" and you're serious about creating such a lifestyle for yourself. How would you go about it?

The basic requirements would be considerable: a true Paleo life would require vast tracts of land and the ability to wander that land unimpeded by fences, highways or people with guns. But it's not at all clear that such land still exists anywhere on the globe. Even our most remote wilderness areas are besieged by people, some of them intent on controlling territory. Small patches of wild land still exist, but they are disappearing fast.

In addition to wild land, you'd also need a tribe to live with. There's really no such thing as "solo Paleo." We can be fairly sure that most primitive peoples stayed with one tribe or another for most days of their lives; it was simply too dangerous to go it alone. So the question presents itself: Can you find a band of men, women and children who'll join you on your Paleo quest? I don't know how it is in your circle, but I sometimes find it hard to get people to go along on an easy day hike on a nature trail, much less a full-time wilderness immersion.

Along with tribe, you'll need an intimate knowledge of your habitat and an oral tradition that goes with it. You can't simply parachute into the wilderness with a knife and a loincloth. Finding food requires deep knowledge of the subtle features of land, plants and animals, and this knowledge resides in the minds and stories of your tribe, especially the elders. Knowledge of habitat is something that is built up over many generations. We simply can't access this knowledge overnight, no matter how noble our intentions.

NEO PALEO

So, if true Paleo is gone forever, what's left for us to do? Modernity as it exists is largely unacceptable; the demands on body and spirit are rapidly becoming intolerable. But if true Paleo is not an option, what are we to do?

The only real alternative is to craft some sort of hybrid that integrates the old with the new, the ancient with the modern. In other words, a neo-Paleo lifestyle.

What would this neo-Paleo lifestyle look like? It's impossible to say for certain. Every person has a unique situation in the modern world and every neo-Paleo life will be a personal creation. In any case, there must be some common themes.

First, there must be a strong emphasis on land and habitat, even if it's just the local park. Yes, we'd prefer a thousand square miles of virgin wilderness, but we'll have to work with what we've got. No matter where you are, get your senses tuned to habitat. Observe the lay of the land and the waxing and waning of vegetation and animals. Walk barefoot whenever possible; use your skin to tell you the characteristics of the earth. You probably won't be able to hunt, but at least you can track. Look for the passage of animals over the land, even domestic dogs and squirrels. Track every living thing in your neighborhood, not just the wild exotics. All life is worthy of your attention and investigation.

Second, start thinking bioregionally. See political boundaries for what they truly are: arbitrary, absurd divisions of land that have nothing to do with biological reality. Focus on the weather, land, plants and animals of your region. Build human relationships that connect with the features of your bioregion.

Next, focus on authentic food. Forget the reductionist's nutrient-by-nutrient breakdown of the modern diet. Instead, look for real food that's minimally processed. Is it recognizable as food? Did it come from a factory or from the land? Would your Paleolithic ancestors recognize it as food? If not, avoid it. If so, consume at will.

If you can't find a tribe of Paleo-savvy people to be with, start building your own. Gather up your active friends and start getting outside. Tell more stories, old and new, play and celebrate together. Create culture.

Whenever possible, go without technological crutches. Choose hand tools over machine tools. Choose land-based navigation over GPS. Choose face-to-face communication over phones and electronics.

Next, focus on frequent, vigorous movement, especially locomotion. Get your body moving. Avoid sports and other movement specializations. Instead, concentrate on the most basic human movement: walking over natural terrain. If that's not enough intensity for you, run like the wind, but do it in harmony with habitat.

As much as possible, get your body in rhythm with natural cycles of light and darkness. Whenever possible, avoid getting up too early or staying up too late. Rely on natural light as much as you can and avoid light supplementation.

Anthropologists have written about "the Paleolithic rhythm," the rough alternation between active hunting excursions and easy days in camp. Many believe that this cyclic activity is fundamentally healthy for the human body. Probably so, but the challenge before us now is to create a neo-Paleolithic rhythm. The ideal beat and timing of this rhythm remains to be seen, but, successful creators will probably develop an alternation between the sedentary digital work that is forced upon all of us and some sort of outdoor movement experience. The details are up to each of us.

THE PARADOX: AVOID THE SEDUCTION

This neo-Paleo challenge is fundamentally paradoxical. On the one hand, we have to recognize and keep conscious the fact that the modern world is constantly trying to seduce us into disordered attention, distraction, physical apathy and ill health. The consumer marketplace is desperately trying to sell us products and services that will pull us into a life of chronic, unhealthy comfort and disconnection with the natural world. To put it bluntly, the modern world is a seduction machine, a porno gallery cleverly designed to appeal to our every desire.

To maintain any kind of Paleo orientation or health in this modern world, we need to develop a powerful inhibition, a neurological counterbalance to the forces of seduction. This calls for a considerable measure of disciplined self-control, powered by the prefrontal cortex of the brain, developed through training. To survive with our health intact, we need to develop the ability to say "No."

At the same time, there's got to be a sensible neo-Paleo balance. Once we've achieved a functional level of inhibition and self-control, there's no reason that we can't appreciate what modernity has to offer our bodies, our health and our happiness. Once we reach a certain level of seduction-resistance, we can enjoy the benefits of modernity.

Yes, the modern world is a distraction machine that will wreck our bodies and torture our spirits, if we allow it. It is also true that the modern world provides wonderful opportunities that can bring us comfort, knowledge and excitement. So expose yourself to the elements, then relish the hot shower, a great meal and a warm bed.

That's the neo-Paleo.

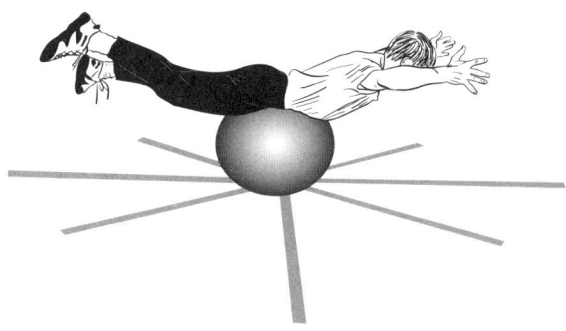

DIGITAL MASTERY

There is something very close to psychopathic about the intrusion of the computer into every conceivable aspect of human affairs.

>   Neil Postman
>   *Teaching as a Conserving Activity*

The real danger is not that computers will begin to think like men, but that men will begin to think like computers.

>   Sydney J. Harris

You are my creator, but I am your master.

>   Mary Shelly
>   *Frankenstein*

You may be surprised to hear this, but I hate my Mac. It has all the things I loathe in a computer. It's fast, has a huge memory capacity and it runs all the major applications smoothly and efficiently. It hardly ever crashes and I can take it everywhere I go. The battery lasts a long time and I can connect to the Internet from just about anywhere.

"So what's to hate?" you're sure to ask. "Isn't this precisely what people are looking for in a computer?"

Actually, the "success" of my computer is precisely what I dislike about it. Not only does it perform the essential functions that I need to make my way in the modern world, it also performs thousands of non-essential functions that I can just as well do without. But it's all so easy, it sucks me into tasks that don't really advance my interests. It keeps my vision centered on a single point in space and keeps my posture in a static position. Worst of all, it keeps me indoors, sapping my vitality and destroying my relationship with the natural world. Slowly but surely, my Mac is killing me.

LABOR GENERATION

Back at the dawn of the digital age, "visionaries" claimed that the computer would be a highly effective labor-saving device that would free us from untold hours of drudgery. No longer would we be shackled to our desks, writing down numbers and words by hand until the middle of the night. We'd be granted a wide-open vista of easy living, free to pursue our favorite leisures, hobbies and fascinations.

Boy, were they off the mark. If the computer is anything, it's a labor-*generating* device, a labor multiplier. By virtue of its multi-function capability, it actually gives us more work to do than we would otherwise have. All computers have done for us is to replace one kind of drudgery with another, less physical form. As computing technology has invaded every last corner of human activity, even the smallest acts of physicality have been stolen from our lives.

Computers remove the body from almost every creative process. I could take notes by hand, but the machine is more efficient. I could make a sketch to illustrate what I'm trying to say, but the machine is faster and more precise. I could walk down the hall and have an actual conversation with a real person, but it's easier to text. Little by little, our bodies are removed from every process. As physicality becomes increasingly irrelevant, we become disembodied and our health and vitality disappear. In the end, the "digital lifestyle" is turning out to be more of a "deathstyle."

AMUSING OURSELVES TO DEATH

It would be one thing if we had the discipline to use our computers as labor-saving tools to streamline our lives and free us to live some authentic dream of true experience. But many of us use computers in the same way we use television, as a tool for escape, avoidance and distraction. As amusement machines, computers pave the way for decreased engagement with the natural world just as they distract us from matters of genuine importance. This is a trend foreshadowed most notably by Aldous Huxley in *Brave New World* (1932), but also by media pundit Neil Postman in *Amusing Ourselves to Death: Public Discourse in the Age of Show Business* (1985).

"SMART PHONES" AREN'T

Of course, no diatribe against computers would be complete without a shot at the so-called "smart phone." According to advertisements, these devices liberate us from our desks and the need to be tied down to any particular place, but this "advantage" seems dubious. Connection to place has been an integral part of human experience for the vast majority of our time on earth. Every primal culture has embedded itself in land and habitat by way of sensation, action, narrative, song and culture. Severing our connection to the land is nothing less than a radical act—an experiment, a shot in the dark. We simply have no idea what "freeing ourselves" from the land will ultimately do to body and spirit. Our surging epidemic of distorted attention suggest we are making a epic mistake.

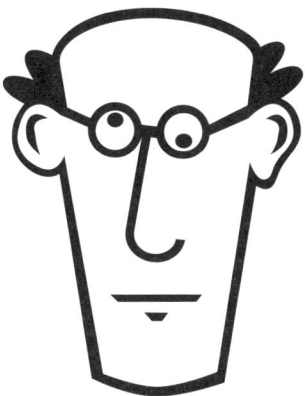

We see the dislocating effects of smart phones and other digital devices in the astonishing inattentiveness of pedestrians and drivers. Cell phone users become nearly blind to their surroundings, oblivious to danger, sight and ambient sound. Texting while driving is now considered a genuine threat to health, linked to striking increases in vehicle collisions. Public health officials have documented an increasing number of cases in which pedestrians have been involved in auto accidents, their spatial and situational awareness blinded by a digital device. Just as the desktop computer sucks the life out of our muscles, smart phones suck the life out of our senses, our awareness of place and our ability to interact with other people in face-to-face settings.

OPPORTUNITY COSTS

Computers are bad enough in what they do to us directly, but they also exact a toll by displacing vital, health-giving life experience. Like junk food that displaces genuine nutrition, computers displace essential human engagement with land, animals and people. Even if computers were entirely neutral in their effect (they are not), they would still harm us by taking us away from our bodies, the natural world and face-to-face interactions with one another.

In the world of economics, *opportunity cost* is the value of the next best alternative that is forgone as the result of making a decision. If, for example, I choose to go to a movie, I cannot spend that time at home reading a book or talking with family and friends.

In choosing a digital lifestyle, opportunity cost is enormous, not just for individuals, but for our society as a whole. We can only wonder about the large-scale use of computers by millions, even billions, of people worldwide: How many trillions of hours of human attention are displaced each year away from contact with other people and the natural world? What are the consequences of displacing human consciousness away from the very things that give us life? What happens to the human mind and body when it stops paying attention to its life-support system? This too is unexplored territory.

RADICAL CLARITY

Of course, this whole discussion poses a nasty conundrum. Computers, for all their body-sucking, health-destroying qualities, are not going away any time soon. Our culture has become so infected with digititis that escape now seems impossible. If we want to get anything done in this modern world, we have to sit down and push the mouse; even the most committed Luddite must spend some time at the keyboard if he is to have any chance of relevance.

It's also the case that, in spite of their proven body-hostile effects, computers do have important and legitimate uses. They are essential for long range connectivity, organizing and logistics. The Internet is obviously a powerful tool for networking by environmental and social activists world-wide. Used sparingly and intelligently, the computer can in fact be a tool to change the world.

And so, it's time to make some hard decisions. What kind of relationship shall we create with these digital tools and machines? As we've seen, the modern computer is a powerfully distractive device that threatens to suck us down into every rabbit hole imaginable. Ultimately, there is really only one way to fight the seduction of the modern computer and that is with *radical clarity of purpose.*

The great thing about knowing our purpose is that it helps us to navigate the computer's many diversions and triage its endless possibilities. Once we know what we really want to create, we can chart a course between trivial pursuits and the digital sink-holes that threaten to consume us.

A sense of purpose also helps us to select the right tools and machines for the job at hand. Intelligent computer use begins, as in all arts, with awareness and intention. It's folly to simply assume that a computer is always the best tool for the job; other possibilities often exist. Power tools are appropriate for some tasks, but hand tools are better for others. Mastery begins when we choose the right tool for the challenge.

So our first task, before we even touch the power button or wake the machine up from sleep, is to refresh our sense of purpose. What is your mission, your goal, your quest? What are you trying to create in this life and this world? What are you trying to accomplish with these immensely powerful tools?

If you don't know, you've got some homework to do. Take a step back from the machine and from the rest of your life and start writing. Clarify your purpose, and do it over and over again. Keep your purpose active and current in consciousness. Refer to it often and use it to illuminate your path through the digital swamp.

And remember this: Your time is precious. Don't give it away to the machine. Reserve your computer time for those projects and tasks that hold some prospect for genuine advancement of your essential interests. Learn the basic skills and apply them intentionally towards your radically clear purpose. Learn the key strokes and find the work-arounds. Buy whatever code you need to make it go smoother, but triage that too.

Advance your purpose, get the word out, promote your cause, and then, as soon as possible, turn off the machine and get back to a healthy human life. It's so much better in the flesh.

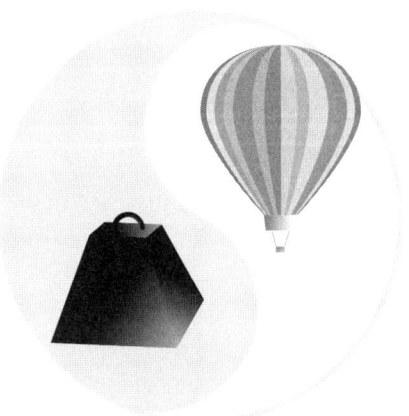

BALANCE GRAVITY WITH LEVITY

Change Your Body, Change the World

COMIC RELIEF

Maybe you're not throwing it right.

> Paula Poundstone in response to the claim that a cat, when thrown into the air, always lands on its feet.

Not living in fear is a great gift, because certainly these days we do it so much. And do you know what I like about comedy? You can't laugh and be afraid at the same time—of anything. If you're laughing, I defy you to be afraid.

> Stephen Colbert

I am not a vegetarian because I love animals; I am a vegetarian because I hate plants.

> A. Whitney Brown

When I tell people that I go to comedy shows and take the expense as a tax write-off, they're usually taken aback. Some of them literally take a step backwards, loathe to be seen in public with such a brazen criminal. Surely my behavior is a stark violation of federal statute or at least a transgression of the public trust. Not surprisingly perhaps, my few remaining friends are either scofflaws themselves or comedians of some sort.

Whether or not my comedy club expense actually qualifies as a legitimate write-off, I have no idea. (None of my friends are IRS agents.) Nevertheless, I propose that the principle is fundamentally sound. After all, I'm working the health beat and stress is a major element in that game. And comedy, especially when it involves the clever re-interpretation of events, is an immensely powerful stress-reducer. I can only wonder and hope that Norman Cousins deducted the cost of his comedy-driven rehabilitation, the source of his landmark book, *Anatomy of an Illness*. If so, he would have established a precedent that may one day keep me free from incarceration.

And besides, if I were to take a $2,000 weekend workshop on "Cognitive re-interpretation of events for professional administrators and health care professionals," the IRS would take no notice. In fact, they'd probably send their agents on all-expense-paid junkets to the very same seminar so that they could learn how to reduce their stress. Then I could rub elbows with the very same people who, in another circumstance, would attempt to destroy my financial life.

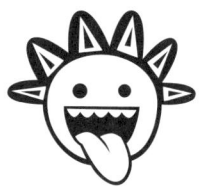

To illustrate my point, let me tell you a story. Lewis Black is one of my favorite comedian-philosophers. Last year, he was scheduled to come to town and I really wanted to see the show. Lewis always finds a way to derail my entrenched ways of thinking. His surprising perspectives open my mind and relax my heart. I laugh long and hard and when I leave the show I'm feeling good. My immune system is running better and my body is moving towards autonomic balance. My biochemical profile is improved and I'll probably require less medical care in the future, thus being less of a drag on an already over-burdened health care system. I'm equally certain that my professional competence, writing and speaking also improve.

So, in anticipation of the event, I called up my friendly health insurance company to check on my policy. Given the powerful benefits of my proposed comedy-health experience, I assumed that they'd jump at the chance to cover the cost of my ticket, but I wanted to be sure. So I spent the better part of my evening waiting on hold and finally, just after midnight, I reached a company rep in Bangalore. In a friendly sing-song voice, she patiently explained to me that in fact, no, my insurer would not be covering my ticket to the comedy show. I was surprised at this turn of events and asked her to double check.

"Well, Mr. Forenziszisic, I am looking at your records and it seems that even if we did cover such, er, procedures, it appears that you have a pre-existing condition that, according to the *Diagnostic and Statistical Manual of Mental Disorders*, invalidates your coverage. Would you like to upgrade your plan? We're running a special this month: your home and all future earnings of you and your offspring, per month, plus your co-pay, of course."

"Er… I had no idea. What are you talking about? I'm in perfect health. I don't have any pre-existing condition."

"Well, Mr. Forexinisxhic, according to your patient records, you are showing a personality disorder characterized by latent fundamentalism, a static worldview and pathological stubbornness. I'm surprised we missed it when you applied. In fact, you never should have been approved for coverage in the first place. You are a statistical error, an anomaly."

I was taken aback, stunned into an unusual silence.

"Er, but wait a second. In the first place, how did you find this out? And in the second place, don't you think that a comedy show is precisely the kind of treatment that would be indicated in a case like this?

"Yes, well, thank you for calling, Mr. Feorgiixzh. We really appreciate your business as a loyal customer. Would you like to participate in a brief survey? It will only take a few hours. Or perhaps you'd like to upgrade to our premium policy? If you'd like, I can transfer to one of our friendly sales associates. Can I put you on hold?"

You won't be surprised to hear that the experience stressed me out and so now I was in a double bind. Not only was my stress level going up, but my health insurer wouldn't pay for the very thing that was most likely to reduce it. It didn't take long for me to conclude that the medical-industrial complex is a vicious circle of pathology; by increasing stress amongst its customers, it simultaneously increases the incidence of stress-related diseases, thereby assuring a constant stream of new business. Somebody is making a lot of money off of highly preventable disease.

THE STATE OF STRESS MEDICINE

But I digress. The point I'm trying to make is that our experience of stress is tightly coupled to our interpretation of events. That is, we now know that events are toxic or beneficial in large measure because of how we frame them.

To understand how this works, we need to understand how stress affects the body. Unfortunately, stress medicine can be a torturous, stressful study in its own right. There's all that biochemistry to learn and then there's the adrenal glands and the hypothalamus and the glucocorticoids (is it adrenaline or epinephrine?) and neurotoxicity and stress-related brain damage and so on. There are thousands of studies and hundreds of books that will either keep us awake at night or put us to sleep in the middle of the day. We could spend years on the subject.

Fortunately, Robert Sapolsky, the rock star of stress science, has boiled the whole complex field down into a simple list that we can read, or if necessary, share with the IRS. In Scientific American, December 2005, Sapolsky writes that individuals are more likely to activate a stress response and are more at risk for a stress-induced disease if they…

- feel as if they have minimal control
- feel as if they have no predictive information
- have few outlets for their frustration
- interpret the stressor as evidence of worsening circumstances
- lack social support

That's it, the entire field in a nutshell. Of course, there are hundreds of animal studies behind each of these statements and miles of supporting evidence to back them up. We can trust Sapolsky. (Anyone who goes to Africa to sit in the bushes and dart baboons with a blow gun to measure their stress hormones is, by my definition, trustworthy. Even better, Sapolsky is a capable comedian in his own right.)

So our experience of stress has to do with our perception of control, predictability, outlets, trends and social support. But few of these are absolutes; most are variable and open to interpretation. As they say, "One man's crisis is another man's play date" and "My best vacation is your worst nightmare." The way we frame an event or relationship can have profound consequences for our stress response. In this way, our personal philosophy, psychology and explanatory style can actually shape the tissue in our bodies. Mind and body are in a constant conversation of reciprocal influence.

Of course, some stress predicaments are straightforward. If a lion chases you up a tree, this is pretty much a compulsory stress event; it's acute and non-negotiable. You can tweak the narrative all you like, but your body is still going to squeeze itself for every hormone and neurotransmitter it can muster. Carnivores are life-or-death animals and they don't have much interest in our personal narratives.

But this is an extreme case and, in the course of a modern human life, an unusual one. In fact, most of our daily predicaments are ambiguous and open to interpretation. That pain in your knee could be a huge stressor if you see it as a threat to your essential running program. Or, it might only be a minor glitch if you decide that it's really an opportunity to go swimming. In this sense, changing your mind might ultimately be one of the keys to changing your body and preserving your health.

FUNDAMENTALISM V. FLUIDITY

In any case, we now know that there's one sure way to position yourself for a chronically activated stress response and that's to adopt and hold tight to a single, static world view. The formula is simple: Develop a perspective on how the world works and *stick to it*. Then, when reality comes barging in with the inevitable counter-argument, you're in for a case of cortisol poisoning and everything that goes with it, including damage to precious blood vessels and neurons.

Heraclitus told us long ago that we can't step into the same river twice; both the river and the stepper are in constant flux. But in a world of uncountable moving parts, fundamentalism attempts to maintain a rigid posture and position. Fundamentalists live in a fantasy universe of static objects, processes and people. When these things behave in ways that deviate from their script, fundamentalists get very unhappy.

It's no coincidence that fundamentalists are almost never funny. They tend to be earnest, stubborn and grim. After all, it's a lot of work, trying to hold the world in one position. And in this state of mind, humor will always come as a threat. As soon as you open your mind to humor, you embrace the possibility of alternate world views. Humor becomes a psychological monkeywrench, an unpredictable and uncontrollable force that threatens to tweak our most cherished assumptions and prejudices.

Ultimately, all fundamentalists have a similar style of relating to the world. Religious fundamentalists, health fundamentalists, cultural fundamentalists, social fundamentalists—all are believers in a static, impossible and utopian universe.

Most of us tend to think of fundamentalists as crazed extremists, zealots and radio talk show hosts who advocate for a single outrageous point of view. But in fact, we're all fundamentalists from time to time, falling into and out of static world views and rigid orientations. It's a trap as old as humanity itself.

The human brain seems particularly vulnerable to the affliction. Changing one's mind can be difficult and challenging work, work that most of us would prefer to avoid. It's far, far easier to simply add more confirming "evidence" that will support one's favorite position.

The paradox is that while fundamentalism aims to protect and defend the self, it ultimately damages that which it seeks to defend. Rigid world views grate up against reality and cause stress, both to the perpetrator and those around him. In small doses, this stress might be stimulating and even productive, but in large doses, it becomes neurotoxic and sociotoxic. This creates a vicious cycle: The stressed-out personality narrows his range of interpretation, action and explanation; his thinking becomes increasingly polarized. But in a complex and fluid world, this black-white orientation ultimately causes more stress, which hardens the personality even further.

THE ANTIDOTE

So what about fear? Most of us would tend to agree with Steven Colbert's claim that comedy displaces fear. But how so?

The first reason goes to simple physiology. Laughter requires that we make an autonomic shift to the parasympathetic nervous system. If we're going to enjoy humor, we have to be in a relaxed, "feed and breed" mode. In this state, oxytocin flows and stimulates human affiliation; we become more receptive to one another. In the process, our sense of humor also acts as a stress barometer: if you can't see the humor in your life or in yourself, then you're probably overdosing on stress hormones. It's time for some kind of a vacation or a change in perspective.

Comedy also gives us a sense of wider possibility and in turn, a sense of control. Instead of becoming trapped within the confines of a narrow predicament, the comedic personality remains fluid and flexible. When demands press in from every direction, humor generates more options for action and resolution. There's less need to fight back with symmetrical power; we remain mobile as our thoughts range over a wider range of territory. In turn, we gain a greater sense of control and the fear, even if legitimate and real, fades in significance.

The power of comedy becomes clear when we think in terms of creativity, limits, borders and boundaries. James P. Carse made this point clearly in his book, *Finite and Infinite Games:* "Finite players play within boundaries, infinite players play with boundaries." Dogmatists and fundamentalists are finite players; they stay within boundaries and defend those boundaries with vigilance. Children, comedians and innovators are infinite players; they play *with* boundaries. In the ebb and flow of a dynamic, chaotic and immensely complex world, finite players will either be eclipsed by events or suffer from stress-related disease as they attempt to maintain their static postures and positions. Infinite players on the other hand, can adapt. If something isn't working, maybe it's time to move the boundaries.

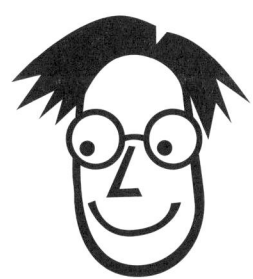

OPEN MIKE

Of course, comedy is not a cure-all for stress or any other of life's predicaments. There are plenty of dysfunctional, high-stress comics who die young, and lots of people use comedy and satire to deepen and harden their fundamentalist beliefs. But nevertheless, in the right hands and with the right spirit, comedy can be an immensely powerful process for transformation, both personal and cultural.

So, if you're in the field of health care, fitness or body arts, go to the comedy shows, keep your receipts and take the write off. Tell your accountant that the expense qualifies as "professional development." When the IRS agents come to your house with a subpoena and a federal marshal, show them this essay. When they're done reading it, ask them how they feel and maybe tell them a few jokes. (Did you hear the one about the IRS agent and the prostitute?) Show them how to reinterpret your tax return and send them away laughing.

If that doesn't work, you might try running.

It's a great stress-reliever.

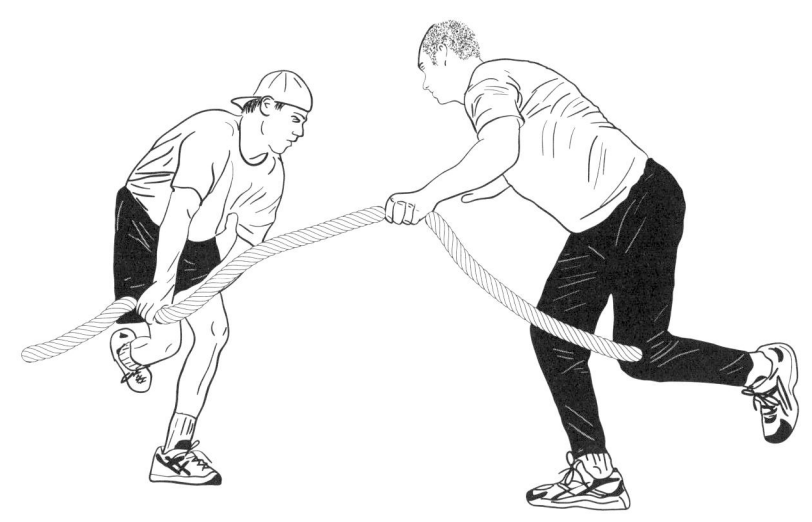

PULL THE ROPE OR LET IT SLIDE
IF YOU HOP, YOU LOOSE

Change Your Body, Change the World

CHANGE YOUR BODY, CHANGE THE WORLD

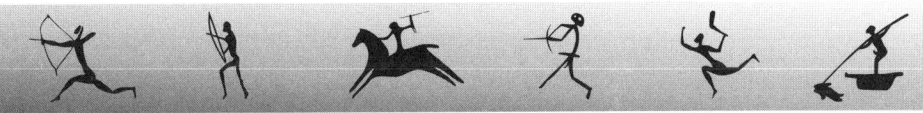

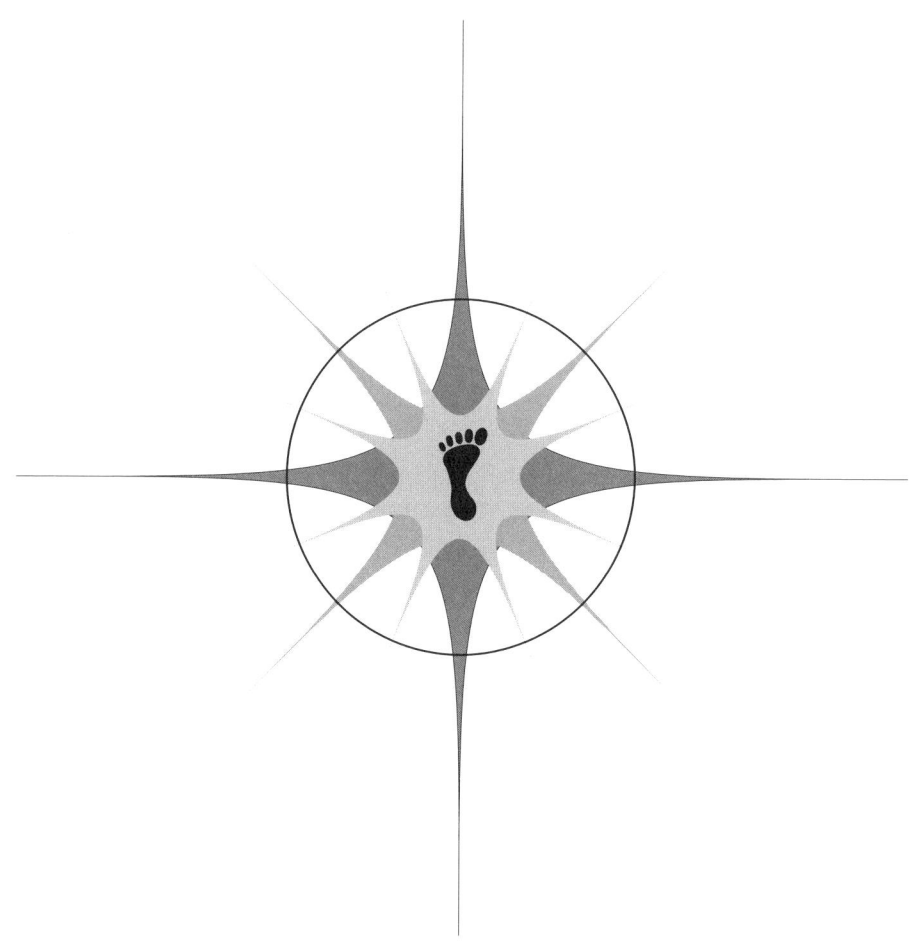

THE FIRST RULE OF NAVIGATION

We have always been taught that navigation is the result of civilization, but modern archeology has demonstrated very clearly that this is not so.

Thor Heyerdahl

I have an existential map; it has "you are here" written all over it.

Stephen Wright

Here's your challenge for today: You're living on a small island in the South Pacific. You and your friends have constructed a small but seaworthy canoe-like craft and loaded it with enough coconuts and tropical fruits to last for many days. Your challenge is to strike out across the open ocean and travel to another island hundreds of miles distant. You must perform this feat entirely without artificial navigation technology; no maps or compass, no radio nav, no dashboard GPS displays in your canoe. In other words, you must make this journey using only your body, your attention and your wits.

If this sounds completely preposterous, consider the skills of ancient Polynesian navigators. Long before the age of map, compass and global positioning technology, Polynesians routinely made long voyages across thousands of miles of open ocean. Aboriginal mariners used their bodies, senses and physical intelligence to get where they were going. They also relied upon knowledge passed by oral tradition from elder to apprentice, often in the form of song. This knowledge base included the subtle qualities of natural features: the motion of specific stars and planet, weather, wildlife, ocean swells and colors of the sea and sky.

The Polynesians were obviously highly skilled and we're inclined to think that they were somehow special, perhaps gifted in some way. But among pre-modern humans, they were not unusual. By necessity, all primal peoples would have been adept at finding their way. After all, their lives depended on knowing their position in relationship to the land. Navigation was routine, as basic to living as eating and breathing.

How else would we have made our way from Olduvai to Patagonia? How else would we have navigated the semi-wooded grasslands of East Africa, the rolling hills of Asia, the outback of Australia and the alpine habitats of Beringia and North America? How many millions of times did hunting parties venture out for days at a time, successfully returning to camp with only their eyes, ears and skin to guide them?

The challenge would have been considerable—many of the bioregions inhabited by primal humans were, to modern eyes, almost featureless. People would have faced thousands of square miles of scrub, marsh, semi-wooded savanna and low rolling hills. Much of this land was the terrain equivalent of the open ocean of the Eastern Pacific: vast, open, dynamic and subtle. But primal peoples managed to navigate it all using only their bodies and extended social intelligence. Sensation, observation, song and story, all in motion, always watching, always mindful and alert to dynamics, change and trends.

WHOLE-BODY NAVIGATION

If you've never been lost, you probably haven't given the predicament much thought. Or, if you have, maybe you just assumed that you'd whip out your smart phone, speed-dial 911 and call in the choppers. If you've got the right hardware and a credit card, you'll be out of the woods and back to a restaurant in no time.

But knowing where you are in relationship to the land is one of the most fundamental aspects of the human experience. It is basic to staying alive, to prospering and even to sanity itself. For most of human history, being lost was just as life-threatening as predators, steep cliffs, lightning strikes and starvation. To be isolated and alone on the mosaic grassland of prehistory would have been a near-death experience or worse.

There's plenty we don't know about the prehistoric lives of primal peoples, but we can be sure of one thing: Paleo peoples navigated their environment using every tool in their mind-body toolkit. They explored, hunted and gathered by vision, sound, odor, texture and the feeling in the soles of their feet. Navigation was completely embodied; it is no exaggeration to say that people used every cell in their bodies to track, monitor and survey their surroundings.

The land was a library that told a story, a story that the human body learned how to read. This was the primal curriculum of land and place. As Jay Griffiths puts it in her book *Wild: An Elemental Journey*, "all landscape is knowledgescape." In other words, there was an intimate continuity between body and land, between flesh and habitat. Land was not "other." Land was us.

Orientation was far more than simply finding a reference point or calculating a set of coordinates. Rather, it was a profoundly psychophysical act, always tied to personal and tribal experience. "I know this valley—this is where we sang for our dying brother." "I know that rock—this is where we found food after a long hunt." "I know that grove— this is where we found the spring with the sweet water." The entire landscape was saturated with story and significance.

A classic example of primal, whole-body navigation is the aboriginal practice of navigation by "songlines." Songlines, also called Dreaming tracks by indigenous Australians, are real-mystical paths across the land which mark the route followed by a 'creator-spirit' during the Dreaming. The paths of the songlines are recorded in traditional songs, stories, dance, and painting.

By using this knowledge, a person is able to navigate the land by repeating the words of the song, which describe the location of landmarks, waterholes, and other natural phenomena. In some cases, the path of the creator-spirit is said to be evident from their marks, or petrosomatoglyphs, on the land, such as large depressions in the land which are said to be their footprints.

For indigenous people, stories were intimately connected to place. One aboriginal elder put it this way in Harvey Arden's *Dreamkeepers: A Spirit-Journey into Aboriginal Australia*. On hearing a request to tell a story out of context he replied, "…those stories are only supposed to be told back where we come from, back in our own country. The story doesn't really mean anything unless you can tell it in *that* place! They're not for reading in a book. They're for tellin' right *there* and nowhere else! They don't make sense anywhere else."

Whether or not you happen to believe in the mystical dimensions of Aboriginal *dreaming*, the fact remains that this system anchored these people to a place, a habitat and a psychophysical home. The strength and power of this connection is simply unimaginable to the modern Westerner. Every detail of the land, weather, vegetation and animal life was integrated into aboriginal bodies, minds and culture. It would not be an exaggeration to say that for these people, land and body were continuous.

DEAD RECKONING

Primal navigation was the norm for the vast majority of human history and only began to give way with scientific developments in the 14th and 15th centuries. Map and compass came into widespread use as Europeans began longer and more audacious ocean voyages. In the process, navigation became increasingly disembodied, most conspicuously with the invention of "dead reckoning." As the name implies, dead reckoning is navigation without natural reference points, striking out into unknown territory with only minimal tools. Just pick a compass heading and travel in that direction for a certain period of time. If you know your starting point, your course and your time, you can calculate your position in two dimensions. You can point to a map and say "I am here."

In dead reckoning, no physical sensations or knowledge of natural features are required. Whether you're aboard ship in a fog bank, piloting an aircraft at night, or on foot in a vast desert, the process is the same: maintain a heading, keep track of time and then calculate. If you have information about wind, current or other natural forces, you can factor these in for greater accuracy, but the primary tools are clock and compass.

In the early years, dead reckoning was a hybrid of sensation and symbols, each supporting the findings of the other. The maritime navigator used maps, instruments and sensation to cross-check and confirm one another, building up a view of position and course. The wise captain didn't entirely trust the new methods, so he always kept a sharp lookout for any possible clues.

Over the course of several centuries however, navigation became increasingly accurate, reliable and disembodied. Physical sensation became less and less relevant to the process. Even worse, sensation came to be seen as a distraction and a potential source of error. As the body was squeezed out, navigation became entirely an abstracted process.

We find the ultimate expression of disembodied navigation in the cockpit of a modern, instrument-equipped, all-weather aircraft and of course, spacecraft. Using a combination of beacons, locator devices and instruments, a proficient pilot can know his location in space at any time, day or night, in any weather conditions. Aside from vision, no physical sensation is required. Aside from a set of eyeballs and a finger to push the buttons, no body is necessary. Instrument navigation is navigation from the neck up.

Over the course of a few hundred years, navigation went from being a highly physical process to an entirely cognitive one. Our native aptitude for sensory observation, attention and awareness of natural features was replaced by "formal operations on abstract symbols."

Today, the disembodiment of navigation is complete. When people are fully outfitted with GPS technology, there is no longer any need for sensation or physicality. Natural cues and features become irrelevant. The position of the sun, the light on the landscape, prominent terrain features, the presence of plants and animals: none of it is important. Just make sure that your battery has a good charge and you're set. Your body and its relationship to the land no longer matters.

THE FIRST THING THAT HAPPENS

There are advantages to technical navigation, of course. By using intelligent devices, we gain speed and accuracy. We also gain scope and panorama; we can navigate distances in conditions that would have been unimaginable in primal eras. We also gain efficiency, predictability and control.

But the downsides of technological navigation are immense and rarely considered. These technologies leave us disembodied, denatured, dependent and detached. When we rely on GPS and similar technologies, we effectively outsource our sensation, skill and judgment. We put our physical sensitivity outside ourselves and hope for the best.

What's the first thing that happens when you master your GPS? Answer: You stop paying attention to the world around you! You give up all concern for reference points, location and position. You could be anywhere and it doesn't matter. Just let the device tell you where you are and where you need to go next. Think of GPS as an anti-awareness technology; once you've got the device, you can put your physical mindbody in idle and check out of the here and now.

DISLOCATION TECHNOLOGIES

Advertisements for "mobile technologies" promise to free us from place, as if our connection to the land was something that needed to be broken, something to be innovated out of our lives. But who among us asked for this convenience? What misguided focus group stood up and said "free us from the land that gives us life?" What market research study concluded that people wanted to be cut loose from their connection to the earth? And if people did in fact ask for this "service," how could they be so ignorant of human biology and history? Where do they suppose that their life comes from?

Separation of people from place is one of the most destructive effects of modern industrial culture. As hundreds of native cultures can attest, divorce from the land is catastrophic for health, community and even sanity itself. We, as dislocated moderns, have lived without a sense of place for so long that we have forgotten its value. Unless we're farming, hunting or fishing, few of us even think of place as having any particular value or meaning; one place is as good as another. As long as there's Internet access and a café, we're content.

There is a powerful irony to this technologically-induced alienation from place. With GPS, we can pinpoint our exact position in an instant. We relax, secure in the belief that we know our location. And yet, in one very important sense, we don't really know where we are. Without some psychophysical relationship to the land, we are, strictly speaking, lost.

"LIVE RECKONING"

The time has come to put down the devices and reestablish a practice of "live reckoning" —a practice that uses natural life and features as reference points for travel. This practice is highly physical and sensation based. Above all, it means paying attention to natural features and natural qualities: natural sight, sound, shape, odor, textures: anything that might give you a clue as to your whereabouts. The key ingredient in is mindfulness: paying attention to subtleties and dynamism of the world around us.

Live reckoning implies a bioregional orientation in which we locate our bodies in relationship to on-the-ground habitat features in the region we inhabit. What, naturally-speaking, is going on in your neighborhood? In your region? Forget artificial political constructs and lines on the map, the national, state and county boundaries that do violence to the land. Focus instead on the watersheds, soils and terrain where you live. Clear your mind of roads, highways and rail lines. Imagine the pre-modern version of your neighborhood. How would you navigate that territory?

THE TERRITORY IS THE TERRITORY

As we practice live reckoning, we become increasingly interested in territory and terrain. Maps and symbols remain useful and interesting, but the real game is on the ground and in the body. In this practice, the live navigator learns to respect the distinction between maps and territory and avoids attaching too much significance to symbols.

The famous expression "the map is not the territory" first appeared in a paper that Alfred Korzybski gave at a meeting of the American Association for the Advancement of Science in 1931. Since then, scholars have referred back to this expression in thousands of ways, mostly pointing to the dangers of careless abstraction. "The word is not the thing itself," they often warn us. You can discuss the symbolic realm all you want, but don't forget that those symbols are unique entities with unique qualities. Symbols are static, condensed, stripped-down snapshots, but reality is rich, subtle and dynamic.

Insightful as Korzybski's phrase was, he was actually late to the game. The ancient Taoist philosopher Chuang Tzu said the much same thing thousands of years earlier, only better: "Words exist because of meaning; once you've got the meaning you can forget the words." Or, "Once you've got the territory, you can forget the map." And the GPS.

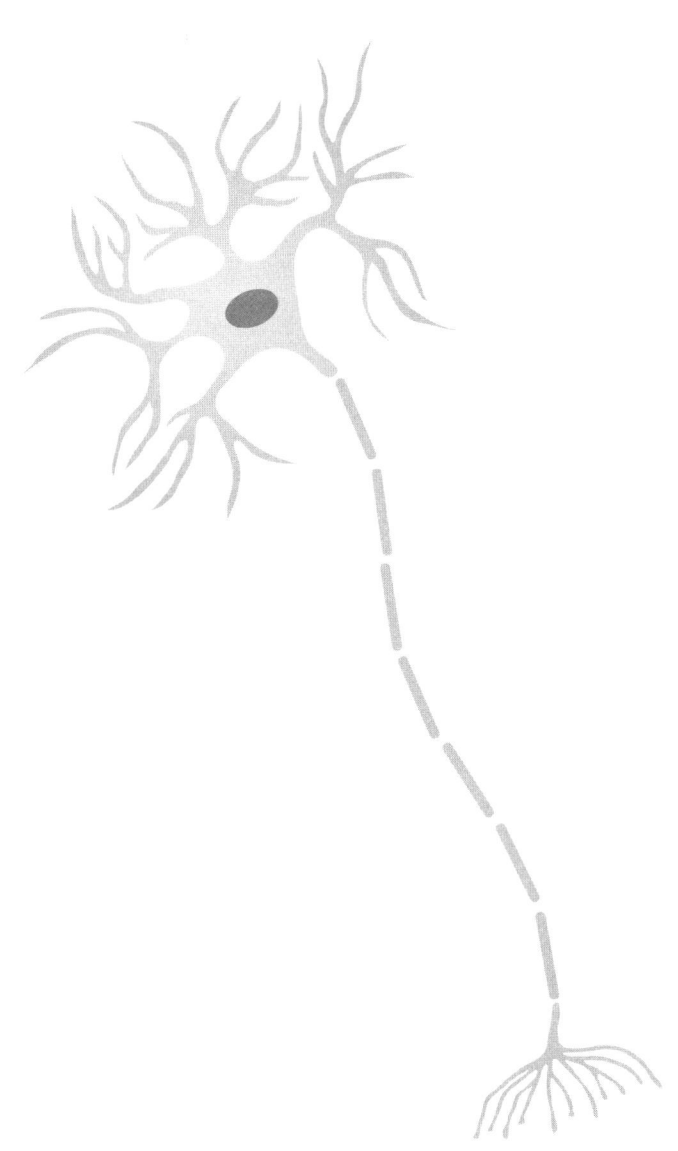

THE FUTURE IS PLASTIC

> I just want to say one word to you. Just one word. Plastics.
>
> Mr. McGuire to Dustin Hoffman
> from the opening scene of *The Graduate*

As students of the human body, we try all sorts of methods to increase our understanding and performance. We read, we train, we go to seminars and listen to one another. These methods all have their merits, but sometimes a story comes along that is so powerful that it transcends our ordinary searching and drives our knowledge to a deeper level in one fell swoop.

One such story comes to us in *The Brain That Changes Itself: Stories of Personal Triumph from the Frontiers of Brain Science* by Norman Doidge, M.D. Doidge is a psychiatrist and a researcher whose primary interest is the plasticity of the nervous system, especially the brain's ability to change, adapt and reorganize itself.

Doidge tells us the story of a neuroscientist and rehabilitation physician named Paul Bach-y-Rita. In 1959, Bach-y-Rita's father, then sixty-five years old, had a stroke that paralyzed his face and half his body. It also left him unable to speak. Experts advised that there was no hope of recovery, but Bach-y-Rita's brother George-then a medical student-refused to accept the prognosis and brought his paralyzed father from New York to Mexico to live with him. He then began a grueling, innovative rehab program.

Fortunately, George knew nothing about standard rehabilitation practices and so began a creative, functional hands-on process of his own. He started with the basics, by teaching his father to crawl. It was a struggle from the very beginning, requiring constant physical support and hands-on attention.

After a few weeks, his father was able to support himself in a crawling position and make forward progress by supporting his weak side against a wall in a hallway. This training went on for months. In addition to basic locomotion, George initiated children's games on the floor, rolling marbles and picking up coins. "Everything we tried involved turning normal life experiences into exercises," he said.

George then began instructing his father in the act of scrubbing kitchen pots in a sort of "wax-on, wax-off" kind of drill. The strong hand holds the pot, the weak hand traces the rim. Over and over, fifteen minutes clockwise, fifteen minutes counter-clockwise. (George was a taskmaster!) The weak arm could scarcely execute the movement, but the rim of the pot gave him a target to focus on.

Little by little, the father's condition improved. Over the course of months, he progressed to the point of standing and then to walking. After about three months, speech started to return and later, a desire to return to writing. At first, he could only use one finger on the keyboard, holding his finger over the desired key, then dropping his entire arm in one crude motion. After learning to control this motion, he learned to drop only the wrist, then just the fingers. Eventually, he learned to type normally.

At the end of a year, his recovery was so complete that he was able to resume full-time teaching at City College in New York. He loved his work and continued teaching until he retired at seventy. He then took another teaching job, remarried and continued working, hiking and traveling for seven more years, eventually dying of a heart attack while climbing mountains in Columbia at 9,000 feet.

If the story ended here, it would be plenty remarkable in its own right. The tenacity, the creativity, the inevitable frustration, the outrageous success in the face of crushing adversity—these are all dramatic elements that deserve our attention and admiration. But for students of the body, the story gets even more interesting.

An autopsy was performed and the son was called to the hospital to review the results. When he arrived, he saw slices of his father's brain spread out on the exam table. After one glance, he was completely astonished. The slides showed an enormous lesion in his father's brain, damage from the stroke that had never healed.

Incredibly, the father's brain had simply bypassed the damaged area and re-organized itself through other neural channels. When pressed to perform new activities, the brain engineered a series of work-arounds, re-routing sensory and motor commands around the damaged area. Cells that had originally performed other functions were recruited to new tasks. Through rigorous training and challenge, the father's brain had figured out a way to re-wire itself.

THE PLASTIC LIFE

The story of Bach-y-Rita's father is breathtaking and inspiring. Clearly, this man was a champion of adaptability, a plastic superhero. But dramatic as it is, this story threatens to obscure the fact that these kinds of plastic changes in the brain are routine and commonplace.

Plastic transformations go on constantly in the human nervous system, especially when we challenge ourselves with new activity. We are forever re-wiring ourselves to adapt to new conditions. For creatures with complex nervous systems, plasticity is the norm. And for primates with over-sized brains, plasticity is a way of life.

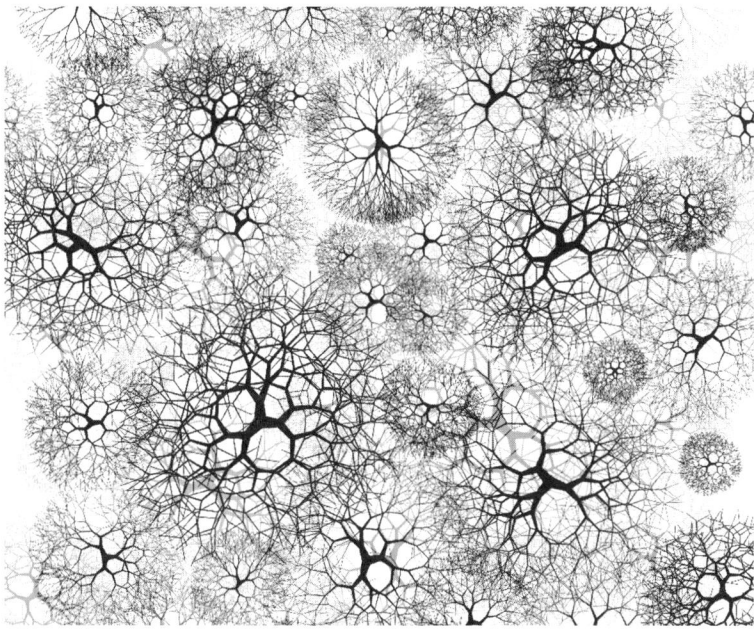

The plasticity of the nervous system is a fascinating study and we could easily get lost in the details. We could even become neural nerds, studying the chemistry of genes, proteins, dendrites and membranes, trying to figure out exactly how plasticity works. But let's forget all that for the moment and bring our attention to the basic experience of living in a demanding, frustrating and challenging modern world.

What really matters here is the life-lesson. In this, the plasticity of the nervous system becomes a metaphor for how we might live better, more functional lives. Suppose that there's an obstacle in your life, a frustration, a stumbling block. You can fight it directly if you choose, but if that doesn't work, you can seek the work-around. Re-wire your perspective and your orientation to some new path.

Suppose you have the equivalent of a "broken blood vessel" in your life, something that causes a "lesion" and a loss of functionality. You've suffered a crisis or loss and now a big piece of your life isn't working. You could dwell on that fact. You could accept the grim prognosis that your situation is static and futile. You could complain and curse your fate. You could give up.

Or, you could start crawling. Get yourself up on all fours and see if you can make it down the hallway. Lean against the wall if necessary. Do it every day. Push yourself. Go right up against your limits. Try new movements and new behaviors. Challenge your brain, your body and your spirit to re-wire itself. Work around the "lesion," whatever it might happen to be. Harness whatever capacities you've got and recruit them into the effort. Take heart in the fact that, as long as you're alive, your body will be looking for a path, a way to generate the action that you're asking it to perform. On any given day, you probably won't notice much of a difference, but after a few months, you'll be up on your feet, walking around and chasing your dreams.

PLAYING IN THE SHADOW OF THE BEAST

> We can no longer afford to delude ourselves, the situation is too critical. Either we put our society on a radically different course so as to reduce its destructive impact on the biosphere, or we delegate this task to the four horsemen of the Apocalypse.
>
> Edward Goldsmith
> editor, *The Ecologist* magazine

I don't know how it is where you live, but I have an immense, ugly animal living in my house. He has a nasty disposition and because he's so big, he monopolizes my conversations and my consciousness. He's a real pain in the ass and I wish that he would just go away. This animal is an enormous bull elephant named "Looming Catastrophe."

Looming Catastrophe is not a furry, feel-good kind of animal. He's a dark, terrifying creature composed entirely of life-threatening trends: economic uncertainty, environmental breakdown, deforestation, population explosion, oil spills, loss of biodiversity, depletion of soil and groundwater, social injustice, racism and terrorism. He's nasty, persistent and demanding. He won't shut up and he won't go away and no matter what I do he's always poking his trunk into everything. He's in my house, in my workplace and in my car. He's on the radio, TV and the Internet. Wherever I go, the elephant goes with me.

The problem with the elephant is that he now disrupts everything in our lives, including our health. Even if he doesn't step on us directly, the elephant interferes with our vitality and our physical happiness. For decades we've been told that the keys to health are diet and exercise. Now we're beginning to realize that the real key to health lies in how we relate to the elephant.

In fact, as the elephant consumes ever more of our attention and psycho-physical resources, the details of sets, reps, carbs and vitamins start to look pretty trivial by comparison. After all, what difference does it make if you tweak your protein-carbohydrate ratio or your training schedule when the biosphere itself hangs in the balance? What good is a beautiful body on an impoverished planet? How does it help to shave a minute off your marathon time when habitat is dying all around us? Who cares if your abs are sculpted when fresh water is disappearing and the oceans are dying?

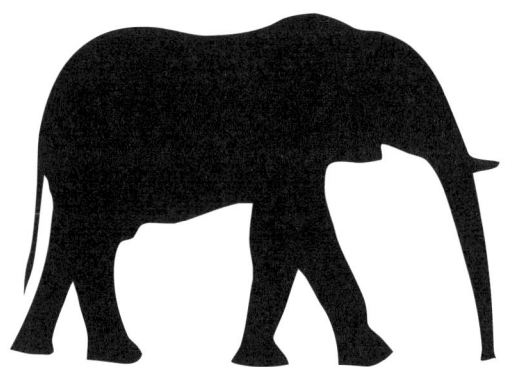

THE POWER OF THE BEAST

"Looming Catastrophe" wrecks our bodies in several ways. In the first place, he's a major distraction. When you've got a nasty beast tromping around in your life, it's easy to get derailed. We spend less time pursuing the things that would normally keep us healthy. We spend less time concentrating on the things that give us joy. The elephant drags us out of our natural play state with the constant threat of disaster.

The elephant also disrupts our neurobiology and in turn our health. The process begins with a sense of anxiety about the future. We feel fear and sometimes outright horror. These feelings of dread aren't just harmless abstractions; they have very real effects on the tissue of our bodies.

When ecologists and biologists talk about "mass extinctions," "ecological overshoot" and "population bottlenecks," we start to take seriously apocalyptic visions of the future. This kind of language even causes us to question our very species-identity. When sober environmental scientists suggest that "we are the asteroid," or "we are a planetary pathogen," we feel a crushing weight of shame.

These catastrophic thoughts and images are bound to stimulate the sympathetic nervous system, even when they're abstract and imaginary. In effect, we respond to the elephant the way we would respond to a real elephant in a wild environment: the body prepares for flight by dumping a powerful cocktail of stimulants into the bloodstream. In an encounter with a real elephant, this neuroendocrine boost saves your life. You run away, climb a tree or dodge the beast. You then return to camp to calm down. Your body weathers the chemical storm and returns to homeostasis. The elephant wanders away and your body gets a chance to rest and repair itself. Your health remains intact.

But our elephant, this "Looming Catastrophe," is a full-time chronic irritant. He stimulates our sympathetic system and keeps on doing it, all day, every day and even well into the night. And every day he keeps getting bigger and stronger and more annoying. And every day, we dump more and more stress hormones into our bloodstreams, preparing to fight or flee.

The effect may be experienced in full awareness, or more likely, it challenges us below the level of consciousness. Our bodies feel the presence of the elephant, even if our minds are engaged with other things. In any case, this chronic state of arousal takes its toll and leads to disease. Living in a state of chronic emergency, our bodies don't have time to repair neurons, vascular cells or vital organs. The end result may come in the form of heart disease, diabetes, strokes or neurodegenerative disorders.

Not only does the elephant wreak havoc with our physical tissue, it also takes an enormous toll on our spirit. Stress wears down our defenses and saps our vitality. We fight to maintain equilibrium, but many of us are dragged down into states of depression. But as we sink, we become even more vulnerable to the elephant and our powers wane even further. This is a classic vicious circle.

Conventional explanations for depression include neurotransmitter imbalances, social isolation, lack of exercise or bad genes. These are genuine factors, but the elephant looms large here as well. The seemingly inexorable rise in depression over the last 50 years may have as much to do with the elephant as anything else. The immense psychic challenge posed by looming catastrophe is particularly threatening to young people. After all, it's hard to be resilient when the future looks grim.

CAN WE CO-EXIST?

Everyone seems to have their own style of dealing with the elephant. Many of us rely on old-fashioned denial. The evidence of looming catastrophe is everywhere and demands our attention, but denialists look the other way. Others see the elephant, but say that it's someone else's problem. "The elephant could never come to our country or our neighborhood. And besides, it's not my job anyway. Don't we pay people to deal with things like this? Dealing with the elephant simply isn't part of my job description. I have other things to do."

Ignoring the elephant may bring a certain level of psychic comfort to the denialist, but it scarcely qualifies as an intelligent response to a planetary emergency. If we are to have any kind of sustainable future or healthy experience in this world, we must keep our eyes open. Denying the reality of the elephant will only make matters worse.

But there's danger in the other direction as well. That is, there's a price to pay for excess vigilance. When we pay too much attention to the elephant, we put our health at risk. The more we read and learn about Looming Catastrophe, the more powerless we feel. Awareness is absolutely essential at this moment in history, but beyond a certain point, excessive attention becomes completely counter-productive.

Given the overwhelming size and nature of the elephant, some of us are inclined to obsess. Knowledge, we believe, is the antidote to our anxiety. And so we study everything about the elephant and its ominous characteristics. If we can just know the facts about climate change, groundwater depletion or species extinctions, we'll be better prepared to act.

But the dose makes the poison. Education is absolutely essential and we would be fools not to investigate the nature of this crisis. But after awhile, we reach a point of diminishing returns. Once the curve tops out, looking at the elephant no longer makes sense. And if we persist, our obsession will ultimately make us sick, rendering us ineffective in our activism.

CREATIVE SELFISHNESS

So how do we act responsibly and intelligently without exposing ourselves to the toxicity of the elephant? Is there a path to health in the midst of this predicament?

As it stands, the elephant threatens to turn us into grim and cynical actors and we run the risk of becoming chronically serious. We fight the beast with determination, but in the process, we begin to abandon the life-affirming behaviors that are so important to our health. We stop taking care of ourselves in subtle ways. We stop playing, we cut back on sleep, we eat faux food; all in the name of bringing more of our serious energy to bear on the challenge of this serious beast.

But this response is backwards. Our predicament now calls for *more* life-affirming behaviors, not less. We need our health now more than ever. Our bodies and our spirits are in grave danger. Turning away from the things that give us life will ultimately lead to even more darkness.

This leads us to a paradoxical formula for success, or at least health and survival. That is, we need to work both sides of this predicament: engage the elephant with intelligent activism and at the same time, pursue more life-affirming behavior. This is creative selfishness, passionate self-care in the midst of immensely challenging circumstance. To remain effective, we need to re-double our efforts at health promotion. We need to spend more time moving our bodies, more time preparing quality food, and more time living in the company of friends and lovers. Save the planet by saving our health and our happiness.

Acknowledge the elephant and fight the beast as best you can. Be a good activist and then forget it. Don't get consumed; build some mental and spiritual firewalls around the beast, then start taking care of yourself and the people around you. Recharge your physical and spiritual resources with all the life-affirming behaviors you can create. The biosphere depends on it.

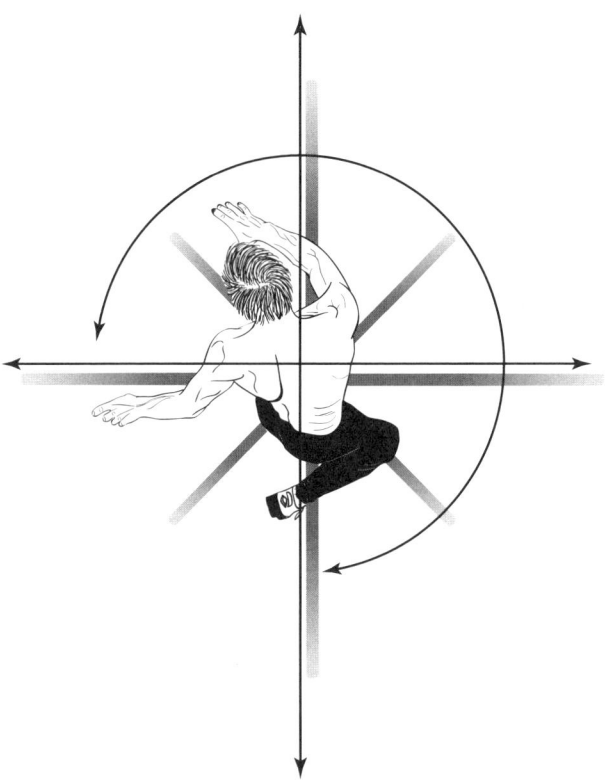

MULTI-PLANE, THREE DIMENSIONAL
REACHES: ONE FOOT

RAPPORT REFORM

> The most effective way to achieve right relations with any living thing is to look for the best in it, and then help that best into the fullest expression.
>
> Allen J. Boone

When we stop to think about the lives of our ancestors and the challenges they faced, we are often struck by a compelling question: how did they manage to stay alive in such harsh conditions?

There they were, naked or nearly so, hungry and defenseless on the semi-wooded grasslands of Africa and Asia. The challenges they faced were raw and utterly immediate. Food was scarce and predators were everywhere. Bad decisions and poor tribal cohesion would have spelled suffering and a high probability of an early death. Margins were thin and extinction was a genuine possibility. So what kept these people alive? How did they manage to survive on that epic migration, all the way from Olduvai to Patagonia?

Anthropologists have a thousand answers of course, but one strikes us as fundamental and particularly relevant to our modern predicament: tribal cohesion. There was something about our human ability to communicate and work together that made survival possible. Social rapport allowed us to hunt and gather in relative safety, to avoid predator attacks, to learn the land and navigate. It also put us on the path to an oral tradition and communal learning, key ingredients that made modern culture possible.

In today's world, our challenges are of an entirely different nature and magnitude of course. No longer do we face the threat of predation or a food supply on the run; many of our challenges are abstract, complex and chronic. Nevertheless, tribal cohesion and rapport are still essential. In a massively complex, interconnected and highly conflicted world, we are in desperate need of social cohesion and interpersonal artistry.

Sadly, our culture has largely forgotten these skills, taken them for granted or simply dismissed them as non-measurable and therefore irrelevant. Interpersonal rapport isn't explicitly taught in schools or the workplace. Aside from common directions to "be nice" and "work together," most curriculums simply bypass the subject entirely. We train people in isolated, singular competencies. We teach young people how to read, write and master narrow specializations, but almost never how to develop rapport in the midst of dynamic relationships. This, of course, is a monstrous oversight and a stark violation of a primary educational objective: to develop well-rounded students.

PHYSICAL FIRST!

So what is the nature of this social cohesion that held primal tribes together? What quality or skill allowed them to agree on anything? How did they reach consensus on where to hunt, where to camp, what to gather and where to explore?

Of course, ancestral tribes didn't all have perfect social cohesion. In fact, they were probably just like us—always breaking up and making up, gossiping, posturing, building alliances and going their separate ways. Surely there must have been diversity among tribes; some were highly cohesive, others fragmented and barely functional. Some had an authoritarian structure backed up by the physical power of the dominant males, while others were more consensual.

But regardless of the diversity and the details, we can be sure of one thing: ancestral tribes created their social life with their bodies, their facial expressions, their posture and the tone of their vocalizations. We moderns tend to forget that social cohesion and rapport is a profoundly physical process. We can talk about the importance of listening, sharing and team-building until our ears fall off, but until we have some physical experience of give and take, of action and yielding, we just aren't going to get it.

ROUGH AND TUMBLE

In the course of normal human development, physical rapport is learned through play, especially rough and tumble play. Young animals learn to experience what action and yielding feel like in their bodies. Their learning becomes deeply ingrained, non-verbal and sub-cortical, which is to say, it becomes extremely influential throughout the course of adult life.

Rough and tumble offers a host of positive benefits. First, it gives young players a sense of what's acceptable and what isn't. It also creates a "safe emergency" that is both stressful and nurturing. This undoubtedly plays a big role in developing and balancing the autonomic nervous system, which is ultimately beneficial for long-term health.

Second, rough and tumble gives players an opportunity to experience and practice role reversals. We see this practice at the dog park every day, especially with younger dogs. An animal may start play in a dominant position, then become submissive in the interest of continuing the play, or vice versa. If you want to keep the action going, you've got to be willing to switch positions quickly and fluidly. "You chase me, then I'll chase you" is a common, unspoken contract. The actual role a player takes isn't nearly as important as the play itself. Obviously, this experience has profound meaning for social function in later life; role fluidity is essential for performance in complex social environments, especially the modern workplace.

Another closely related quality that's developed in rough and tumble play is "self-handicapping," the intentional withholding of physical power in the interest of continuing play. This is commonly observed in dogs, cats, primates and other mammals. Larger and more powerful animals often turn down their intensity so that play can continue. This too has enormous potential in adulthood: animals that learn to self-handicap can adjust their powers to suit conditions. This skill can help to preserve motion in relationships of all kinds.

MIRROR MIRROR

In addition to rough and tumble play, we also develop social cohesion and rapport through the mirror neuron system. To make a long story short, mirror neurons are brain cells that fire both when observing or producing movement. The mere act of watching another person performing a movement sets off a cascade of neural activity in our brains and bodies. When we watch other people move, we effectively run a simulation of that movement in our own bodies. This gives us a chance to feel what other people are feeling in a direct and intimate way. Not only is the physicality of others highly contagious, it also serves to spread emotion and meaning through the tribe.

Neuroscientists are fascinated by mirror neurons and now believe that they are the foundation for many social processes, including empathy. When others move their bodies in our presence, we get an intimate sense of their inner experience. Of course, for this system to work, you actually have to spend time in the presence of real people who are moving their bodies in meaningful and appropriate ways. Real-time, face-to-face interactions are essential.

CONSEQUENCES OF APHYSICAL EDUCATION

Sadly, this brings us around to the disturbing reality of modern curriculums and the immensely destructive consequences of aphysical education. By taking the body out of schools and the workplace, we've discarded the very experience that holds the most promise for solving social and relationship problems.

When people are deprived of rough-and-tumble play or other rapport-building physical experience, human relationships almost inevitably become distorted. Unfamiliar with the give and take of vigorous physical play, people drift off to one pole or the other: becoming passive, aggressive or chaotic and unpredictable.

Play deprivation, whether imposed in the home or by institutions, is serious business with serious consequences. When we deprive young animals (and children) of play, we are likely to see some or all of these downstream effects: inability to establish and sustain rapport, inability to converse in meaningful ways, lack of behavioral flexibility, rigid, fixed social roles and attention problems.

Sadly, we make matters even worse by our choice of games in modern education. Even when we do offer physical opportunities, we institute competitive, zero-sum sporting contests. In these events, the ultimate objective is victory over an opponent, a context that rewards power, control, strength and cunning. Some rapport-building is possible under the heading "teamwork," but this is simply a means towards a competitive end. Professionalized youth sports add to the problem by training children to adopt fixed roles and positions on their teams; instead of learning behavioral flexibility, these players learn rigidity.

Not only do we deprive children of rapport-building rough and tumble play experiences, we also deprive ourselves of essential mirror neuron experience. For millions of years, conversation and communication between people has been synchronized in real time. Messages were shared across common physical experience. I could watch your body as you talked to me; you could watch my body as I listened. This generated an immensely rich flow of information, both verbal and non-verbal. Actual words were backed up by tone of voice, speed of delivery, facial expression, gesture, posture and eye movement. Communication was holistic.

But now, in our headlong rush for efficiency, we've chosen to take the body out of the process. First with telephones and now with electronics, we've created communication patterns that are completely asynchronous and alien to the human experience. If I send you an email, I not only strip my communication of essential non-verbal meaning, I am also forced to wait an unknown period of time for a reply. During the interim, our bodies are completely invisible to one another and communication ceases. The reply, when and if it comes, is likely to sound like a *non sequitur*, an isolated string of characters that must be decoded to be understood. Naturally, this leaves my mirror neuron system completely out of the picture. Even worse, it can lead to a cascade of misunderstandings.

Ultimately, the consequences of our aphysical and competitive social education are felt in almost every dimension of our experience. Without a positive physical-social experience to draw on, people fail to learn the fluid give and take of rapport. And without a sense of rapport, people become bad conversationalists, bad musical partners, bad dancers, bad business partners and of course, bad lovers and bad spouses.

Consider the bad conversationalist. This person has no sense of give and take, no sense of rhythm and no sense of sharing. He either talks incessantly or not at all. He makes no attempt to find out what we think about things, or he pumps us for every detail. He interrupts conversations at random, entirely without awareness. His stories go on for eternity or fizzle out without a point, lesson or climax.

Bad dancers and business partners are just as annoying. Unschooled in the fundamentals of physical give and take, they either advance or retreat compulsively. They take a position and hold fast, terrified of movement, dynamism and uncertainty. Instead of adjusting to the play, they fight, run or freeze, wrecking the movement and possibly the relationship as well. The same goes for bad lovers and bad spouses, only more so.

REMEDIAL ED

So the time has come for some remedial education in rapport. How do we do it?

Obviously, words can only do so much. Instead, the process has got to be experiential. We've got to get the physical body in on the action. Ideally, this physicality should be social and playful, with an emphasis on real-time, whole body communication.

For those who missed out on rough and tumble play in their youth or who've forgotten its lessons, we need a creative approach. Not many adults are willing to get down on the floor and wrestle freely with one another, no matter how promising the payoff. Adults like to believe in their sophistication. They may very well wrestle with their grandkids, but not one another.

Nevertheless, all is not lost. We can keep physical social play alive with dance, martial art and even massage and theatre. Depending on the enthusiasms of the group, we can invent games that put people into proximity to one another. Physical contact is best, but even the simple observation of other human bodies in motion is enough to turn on the mirror neuron system. This will promote rapport and empathy.

EQUIPOISE

For young and old alike, the challenge of rapport ultimately inspires us to develop a sense of *equipoise*, the state of being balanced or in equilibrium. The standard definition of equipoise speaks of "equality in distribution, as of weight, relationship, or emotional forces; equilibrium," but I prefer to think of *equipoise* in terms of its full psychophysical potential: a person's willingness to move in any direction at any time, either advancing or retreating to maintain movement and develop rapport. It's a willingness to sculpt and be sculpted, act and be acted upon, to lead and be led.

When we're in equipoise we are without an overt agenda. Instead, we stand ready to create in process, in time and in relationship. The Chinese would say that we're poised between yin and yang; we hold both potentials at the ready. In equipoise, we're in the sweet spot between acting and listening to the world.

Equipoise is an ideal psychophysical state, perfect for athletics, dance, relationships and business. It gives us the potential to move, to adapt and revise as conditions change. Even better, it is profoundly educational. By coming to a relationship in a balanced manner, we can either teach or be taught.

RAPPORT WITH THE WORLD

Physical rapport with others is obviously an essential skill, but it's only a beginning, a model for rapport on other levels and with the world at large. Rapport and equipoise are fundamentally about relationship, and this can be *any* relationship, including our relationship with the land, with nature, with culture and with ourselves.

The same principles apply in every case. When looking for rapport with culture, move with equipoise. Be a give-and-take participant; act upon culture to advance your creations, but be willing to be moved by it as well. When looking for rapport with nature, exert power and control as necessary to survive, but retain your willingness to be moved, to listen, to be taught. When looking for rapport with self, be neither adversary nor victim. Touch the other side of yourself as a rough and tumble play partner. Wrestle with abandon, reverse roles as necessary and whatever you do, keep the play going.

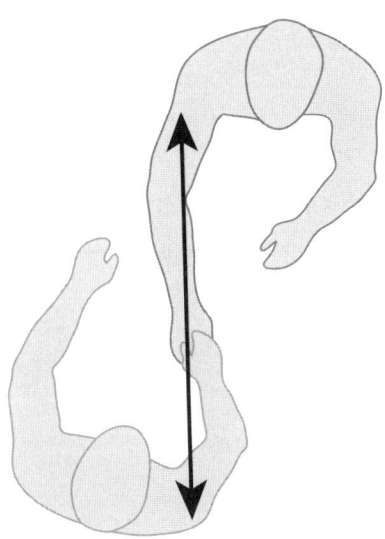

PARTNER-RESIST
LINEAR STROKE, USE HIPS AND CORE
SMOOTH RESISTANCE

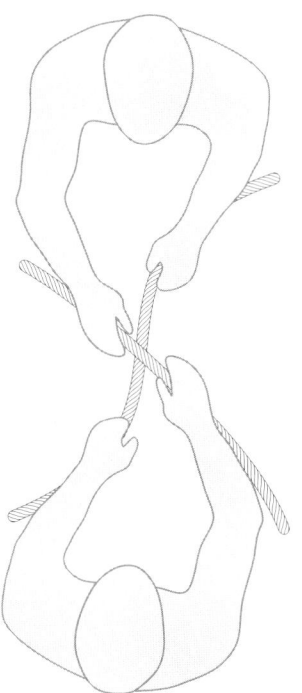

PARTNER-RESIST:
GIVE YOUR PARTNER SMOOTH RESISTANCE,
USE YOUR HIPS AND CORE

Change Your Body, Change the World

EMBODIED SOLUTIONS

> Watching a child makes it obvious that the development of his mind comes about through his movements... Mind and movement are parts of the same entity.
>
> Maria Montessori, 1967

> What makes my Thinker think is that he thinks not only with his brain, with his knitted brow, his distended nostrils, and compressed lips, but with every muscle of his arms, back and legs, with his clenched fist and gripping toes.
>
> Auguste Rodin, 1840-1917

If you ever get a chance to visit an elite athletic training facility, be sure to watch the senior coach or head trainer. Look for an older guy in a baseball cap, a guy who's strong and vigorous, but with some mileage on his body. He carries a clipboard, but doesn't look at it much, preferring to keep his attention focused on his athletes. It won't be long before you hear him yell out instructions that sound like this:

"Lift the weight with your whole body!"

"Integrate! Spread out the forces."

"It's all one muscle!"

"Keep relaxing; let the chain do the work."

"Toenails to fingernails!"

Our coach is practicing a holistic philosophy of movement, a functional, whole-body approach to athletic development. He knows from experience that this method works; not only does it improve performance, it's also aesthetically pleasing and intellectually fascinating.

But if the elite athletic coach advocates a whole-body approach for sports performance, why shouldn't we use a similar philosophy in the world of education and decision making? How might it work in the world of business? Just imagine a management coach using similar language. How would this sound in your office?

"Make the decision with your whole body!"

"Integrate!"

"Keep relaxing, let your entire being find the solution."

"Toenails to fingernails!"

Welcome to *embodied cognition*, the ancient yet revolutionary idea that mental processes are not just of the brain, but of the body as a whole. This post-Cartesian concept is about to turn the worlds of education, management and life arts upside-down. The study of embodied cognition is about to get very interesting and for some parts of our culture, very inconvenient. Embodied cognition will shake things up across the landscape of education, management, business and psychology.

But what exactly is embodied cognition? The basic definition holds that the human mind is determined by the form of the body—ideas, thoughts, concepts, categories and all other aspects of the mind are shaped by the body. But it's not just physical form that shapes our cognition, thoughts and decisions; it's our entire physical experience. In *Embodied Cognition: A Field Guide*, author Michael L. Anderson puts it this way:

> Instead of emphasizing formal operations on abstract symbols, the new approach foregrounds the fact that cognition is, rather, a *situated activity*, and suggests that thinking beings ought therefore be considered first and foremost as acting beings.

Taken together, these definitions tell us that intelligence is not simply concentrated in the head and the brain. Rather, it's distributed throughout the body and across the body's relationship with the world. Furthermore, cognition is a collaborative, conversational process: we think with our brains, our bodies and our physical experience in motion.

For many of us, this entire proposition comes across as completely self-evident. "Well, yeah, Dr. Obvious. You say that the mind is embedded in the body? You want a Nobel prize for *that*? Maybe you ought to talk to a dancer or a surfer."

After all, most of us have direct experience with the mind-body connection as it relates to problem solving, outlook and decision making. Even the dullest among us has struggled with an intractable problem and then gone out for a run, only to watch in amazement as the problem that was formerly impossible now solves itself. Many of us have discovered that dark moods and rumination magically fade away after a good romp in the gym or the woods. People have known about the mind-body connection for a very long time.

But the Cartesians are an extremely stubborn lot and need to be convinced, preferably with stacks of neck-up data. Naturally, if we ask a cross section of sedentary intellectuals about embodied cognition, they'll be skeptical. They'll say it's an idea that needs more testing and research before we can take it seriously. But of course they would say that; embodied cognition only seems revolutionary to people with no physical experience to draw upon.

Not only does embodied cognition make sense to the physically literate, it also makes sense in terms of human evolution. Natural selection, after all, acts on whole bodies; it's the whole animal that either makes it to reproductive age or doesn't. Selection pressures such as food shortages, disease and predators act upon whole organisms. Flesh, emotion and executive brain function have always combined to make decisions about behavior: where to hunt, when to run, fight or flee. In other words, embodied cognition is the historical norm for humanity.

And it's not just humans either. Primatologist Frans de Waal made this telling observation after decades of working with chimpanzees and other primates:

> To learn from others, apes need to see actual fellow apes: imitation requires identification with a body of flesh and blood. We're beginning to realize how much human and animal cognition runs via the body. Instead of our brain being like a little computer that orders the body around, the body-brain relationship is a two-way street. The body produces internal sensations and communicates with other bodies, out of which we construct social connections and an appreciation of the surrounding reality. Bodies insert themselves into everything we perceive or think. (Discover Magazine, Oct. 2009)

THE POWER OF EMBODIMENT

The field of embodied cognition is set to explode with new ideas of brain-body interaction. In the meantime, we already know an enormous amount about the virtues of embodiment and how physical experience promotes better brain function.

We know that physical movement (exercise) decreases stress hormones and in turn facilitates improved decision making. It also promotes neurogenesis, the growth of new brain cells, and the production of neurotrophins, substances that promote the growth of dendritic branching. We also know that an active lifestyle correlates with higher intelligence and better cognition.

Dr. John Ratey makes this point abundantly clear in his book *Spark: The Revolutionary New Science of Exercise and the Brain*. For Ratey, there is a "…direct biological connection between movement and cognitive function…exercise is the single most powerful tool you have to optimize your brain function." It is now becoming clear that physical movement is more than just a way to optimize health; it's an essential element in management, planning, administration and decision making. Managers who fail to use physical movement in their practices are using only partial intelligence; the decisions that they produce will be sub-optimal at best.

NATURAL COGNITION

Movement and exercise have powerful effects on the brain and decision making performance, but there's more to being embodied than just moving and feeling our limbs. There's also context, and that means nature.

Given what we know about human history and the fact that our ancestral physical experience took place in natural environments, we can safely suppose that cognition is also a conversation between mind, body and nature. Just as people are increasingly aware of embodied cognition, we are sure to see an upsurge of interest in *natural cognition* as well.

Richard Louv gives us a sense of this mind-nature connection in his book *Last Child in the Woods: Saving Our Children From Nature-Deficit Disorder*. He points to a cluster of symptoms that are associated with isolation from the natural world: trouble paying attention, listening, following directions and focusing on tasks. His primary focus is on children, but we can bet that these patterns of disordered attention plague adults as well, and for similar reasons.

For example, Louv cites a study presented to the American Psychological

Society in 1993. Stephen and Richard Kaplan surveyed more than 1,200 corporate and state office workers. Those with a view of trees, bushes, or large lawns experienced significantly less frustration and more work enthusiasm than employees without such views. In another study, researchers compared groups on proof-reading performance. The group who backpacked in a wilderness area showed better performance than those who traveled to an urban area or who took no vacation. Other studies show additional benefits to "green" exposure: better motor coordination, increased ability to concentrate, less impulsivity and improved ability to delay gratification. The same effect applies to mammals, primates and rodents across the board: environmental enrichment increases brain activity, just as environmental deprivation actually shrinks the brain. The effect is well understood by neuroscience: environmental stimulation leads to thicker myelin sheaths, which allow neurons to fire more efficiently.

None of this comes as any great surprise, of course. The brain, like the body, evolved over the course of millions of years, nearly all of that time in natural environments. It makes sense that our cognition would be highly attentive to natural shapes, sounds, colors, textures and forms. After all, our lives depended on it. Brains that failed to attend to natural qualities were unlikely to make it to reproductive age. And now, when we take away natural shapes, colors, textures and forms, the brain gropes for connection. If it comes up empty, attention becomes disordered and the spirit becomes depressed.

Nature not only make our bodies feel better, it also gives us wonderful raw material to think with. It provides us with primal forms, patterns and structures. It gives us a sense of dynamism, rhythm, pace and place. These lessons can in turn be applied to any form of decision making in any realm.

The effect becomes even more profound with vigorous physical movement. People who move their bodies in outdoor settings expose themselves to more of Nature's content. Natural qualities are welcomed by the senses and are absorbed more completely.

In this way, the natural world teaches us not just how to move, but also how to think. People who move their bodies in outdoor settings are more likely to think organically and systemically. They are less likely to fall into reductionistic habits of thought and are more likely to look towards integration, harmonies and connection. This organic outlook is powerful medicine for all decision makers, especially those who are forced to work in abstracted, non-natural realms of thought and action.

DANGEROUS PEOPLE

The benefits of embodied, natural cognition are clear, but the broader implications can be disturbing. Given what we know about the tight integration of the human body and the positive effects of movement in nature, we begin to wonder about the abilities and decisions of disembodied, denatured people in positions of power.

With this in mind, I would like to offer some blunt opinions about disembodiment in the modern world. I come to these opinions with my tongue slightly in check, but only slightly. There is a subtle reality here, one that we must take seriously. That is, if embodiment is in fact a path to better decision making and intelligence, then we ought to treat disembodiment and denatured living as a genuine threat to public health and welfare.

The first conclusion is simple: sedentary people are dangerous. Because they traffic almost entirely in formal operations on abstract symbols, divorced from body, emotion and nature, they are capable of almost any error. Abstract symbols have no physical or emotional content; they are bloodless, breathless and soulless. Because they have no connection to body or land, we forget their meaning and their gravity. When sedentism becomes extreme, the world becomes increasingly theoretical. And when the world becomes theoretical, decisions lose their significance.

Inactive people are also suspect because they are more vulnerable to the corrosive decision-warping effects of stress. Because they fail to pump their bodies, sedentary people tend to fester in a stew of adrenaline and cortisol. In the sort term, this drives them towards action—action which may or may not be truly necessary. And in the long term, stress hormones tend to shrink the prefrontal areas of the brain that are responsible for impulse control and emotional regulation. This leads to short-term thinking and failure to see the big picture.

Just as disembodied people are dangerous, so too are nature-deprived people. Given what we know about the role of the natural world in supporting human health, denatured cognition simply cannot be trusted to make good decisions. Those who fail to make contact with the natural world lack a powerful source of inspiration, metaphor and imagery. This leads to poor cognitive performance and in turn, poor decision making ability.

The bad decisions that flow from a neck-up thinking style have personal consequences to be sure, but they also ripple throughout our social and environmental lives. With billions of people making hundreds of decisions every day, even subtle levels of disembodiment and denatured living can have profound consequences for communities, cultures and the biosphere as a whole. Living a disembodied and denatured life is not just bad for individuals, it's bad for everyone.

EMBODIED SOLUTIONS

So what are we to do with our disembodied minds and our sedentary, denatured bodies? How do we re-create an integrative, whole-animal experience? How can we enhance our decision-making skills by using our entire mind-body-experience?

The short, simple answer is to start with *any* kind of physical experience. Stop searching for elite programs, professional trainers and highly specialized disciplines. Instead, get moving by any means possible. Our immediate objective is embodiment, not athletic excellence. So, it's all good: physical labor, massage, sex, art, play, cleaning out the garage, walking the dog. Barefooting is particularly valuable as it delivers more sensation than just about anything else.

Of course, all other things being equal, vigorous is better. The goal is to increase our sense of physicality and this calls for effort, immersion, commitment and engagement. To really embody your experience, you've got to get into it, and that means pushing yourself outside your comfort zone, especially if you've been sedentary for a long time. In this quest, there is simply no substitute for authentic, full-body participation; the goal is to feel your physical self, striving at the limit of sensation.

The smartening effects of cardiovascular exercise are well-established. We know that vigorous regular movement contributes to creative problem solving. We need to get the heart rate up, and keep it up, in a sustained, powerful effort. When the sweat begins to flow, the brain begins to grow.

Clearly, decision makers need to be doing more heavy breathing, growing their brains and sharpening their intelligence. But there's more to this story. The next frontier in decision making and cognitive enhancement will be the practice of diagonal, spiral and circular movements. Multi-plane movements are great for athletic development *and* cognitive development. Twist your body, rotate across the center line and you'll stimulate your brain in an entirely novel way. If you want to think three-dimensionally, it helps to move three-dimensionally.

And naturally, Nature. Get out of the big box office and the big box gym. Engage and embrace the elements. Grow your brain by observing, listening and witnessing natural growth. Move your body in public parks, in wilderness areas and in the gaps between urban dead zones. Improve your cognition with natural sensation. Replenish your mind and body with primordial sights, sounds and textures.

EMBODIED TALK

As our understanding of embodied cognition becomes more complete, we'll begin to change both our behavior *and* our language. The common phrase "Let's sit down and think about this…" will become begin to sound increasingly untenable, even absurd. We'll see it as a call for a disembodied half-effort, one that sets the stage for an incomplete, possibly misguided solution. Ultimately, we'll become skeptical of all sedentary decisions, recognizing them as ineffective at best and dangerous at worst.

Our new language will integrate movement and cognition into an increasingly comprehensive practice. We'll begin to show new respect for active cognition and recognize it as a more integrated, practical and effective solution. Our talk will reflect this new appreciation. We'll say "Let's take this problem out for a run." Or, "Let's walk with this for awhile." "Can we dance with this and see what we get?" Translation: "Let's bring our whole bodies to bear on this problem."

The time has come to take our talk seriously. Next time you're pondering your personal challenges, managerial dilemmas or the human predicament at large, resist the habitual urge to "sit down and think about it." Instead, bump your cognition up to the next level with movement in natural surroundings. As the Barefoot Sensei advises, "Take your thinking out for a run." Or, as the athletic coach might tell say:

"Make the decision with your whole body."

"Integrate!"

"Keep relaxing, let your entire being find the solution."

"Toenails to fingernails!"

It works for athletes and it can work for us too.

RUT CRAFT

Routines and habits are the Known, protecting us from the Unknown. Habits are also called home. Habits tame the raw wilderness of existence into the civilized comforts of everyday life. Unfortunately, as we all know, habits gradually domesticate all the wildness and energy out of life. So much energy gets bound up in routines and habituated patterns, keeping them alive, that your life goes dead instead. Thus, if you want to discover again the wild side of life, you have to leave "home;" you have to break or dissolve your habits in order to release the energy locked up inside them.

> Ed Buryn,
> *Vagabonding in the USA*

As a single footstep will not make a path on the earth, so a single thought will not make a pathway in the mind. To make a deep physical path, we walk again and again. To make a deep mental path, we must think over and over the kind of thoughts we wish to dominate our lives.

> Henry David Thoreau

New planets require new habits.

> Bill McKibben
> *Eaarth: Making a Life on a Tough New Planet*

I used to think that I had free will. I imagined myself as an independent animal, a free agent traveling the world with conscious intent and focused, intelligent action.

Boy was I ever wrong. As I got older, I began to realize that a lot of what I was doing each day was the product, not of intentional deliberation and intelligence, but of routine and habit. You're no doubt familiar with the usual suspects: sloth, over-eating, sloppy conversation, robotic relationships, habitual movement patterns, cookbook training. Same breakfast, same route across town, same run, same workout, same patterns of speech, same aisle in the bookstore, same habits of posture, same cognitive ruts, same emotional reactions to my predicaments.

On some days, I feel as if I'm a slave to my compulsions, a victim of the grooves that are etched in my brain. It also seems that some of those grooves are leading me inexorably towards those ever-popular seductions: sugar, fat, alcohol, sloth and reality TV. Fortunately, I am usually rescued from that fate by another, more powerful set of habits that steer me towards vigorous outdoor movement, social play and physical happiness. Decades of training in sport and martial art has given me a set of body-friendly, life-promoting behaviors to fall back on. But still, this ongoing conflict between habits makes me wonder how different things might be if my ruts and routines were to take me in another direction. Who's in charge of my health and indeed my life anyway? Is it me or my habitual behavior?

Herein lies the pivotal issue in the world of health, lifestyle and fitness. The problem of modern health is not so much that people lack facilities, expert knowledge or access to trainers and coaches. Rather, it's that they're trapped in patterns of living that progressively destroy their health. Too many bad habits, not enough good ones; it's a familiar, boring story. If we could figure out how to re-wire our habitual behaviors, getting in shape and staying healthy would be a relatively easy matter.

Not only are habits a powerful force in individual health, they also play out in our relationships to one another, our culture and the natural world at large. Patterns of dysfunctional relationship, environmental apathy, social injustice and ignorance are just that, patterns. Most of us relate to the wider world, not out of conscious intention, but out of cultural routine. Habitual thinking and behavior even spans generations, with profound, unconscious consequences. Cultural habits do to the earth and society what individual habits do to the body.

Habits are so profoundly influential over the course of our lives that we might suppose that health and life education would include intensive training in "habit education," the recognition, adjustment and revision of habitual behaviors. After all, if you know how to adjust your habits, everything else about health and life should eventually fall into place.

Unfortunately, this is not what we see. The boilerplate prescription for health and fitness tells us what to eat and how to move, but that's usually the end of it. In fact, the fitness industry is itself profoundly pro-habitual: the same workout and nutrition advice repeated *ad nauseum* in every publication on every newsstand across the land. Sadly, habitual advice is unlikely to be a solution to habitual lives.

So, let's have a look at ruts, routines and habit education. What good are habits anyway and what are we going to do with them?

THE BRAIN IS A HABIT-FORMING ORGAN

Like almost everything else in the human experience, it all starts with the brain—specifically, the nervous system. This incredible system runs the entire mind-body show. It brings the far-flung outposts of the body into conversation with one another so that they can regulate each other's activity. It senses, it integrates, it drives movement and behavior, but most of all, it forms patterns of connectivity. Like an enormous tree in a topiary garden, the brain is constantly in the act of growing dendritic shoots, reaching out in an attempt to connect itself with the rest of the body. Branches that get used tend to remain in place and become stronger. Branches that go unused tend to atrophy and disappear. A neural etching machine, the brain continually creates patterns of thought, perception and action, deepening patterns that are used most frequently.

Neuroscientists describe this process of learning and habit formation as "use-dependent plasticity." They even give us a snappy catch-phrase that etches itself into our minds and memory: "neurons that fire together tend to wire together." The specifics are fascinating, but for the moment, not particularly important. What is important is the fact that the brain is continually re-creating itself in response to use. Circuits that are used become stronger, circuits that go unused become weaker. This process deepens our inclination to do more of what we've done in the past. Our brains and bodies are always forming habit.

In essence, the functional unit of the nervous system is the *groove*. This informal term refers to any learned, habitual pattern of activity in the nervous system. Thus, one of the fundamental challenges of living in the human body comes down to this: grooving and ungrooving our brains, bodies and behavior.

The raw material for this process is reps. It makes no difference what the context is: repeated use of the nervous system, in any form, increases the chances that such an action or behavior will be repeated. We can talk about musical reps, aerobic reps, kettlebell reps, emotional reps, conversational reps or interpersonal reps; it makes absolutely no difference. The greater the number of repeated efforts, the deeper the groove, for better or for worse. Ultimately, practice makes permanent.

Given our obsession, preoccupation and embarrassment over our dysfunctional habits, many of us will be inclined to say that all habits are bad. But habits, ruts and routines are actually essential for learning, survival and performance; they allow us to do things faster and with less conscious attention over time. Habits are, in effect, labor-saving creations of our nervous systems.

Neural grooves are immensely valuable to any organism that wants to succeed in a complex environment. Once an action or behavior is etched in or learned, neurological resources are freed up to meet new challenges. Once we learn to walk, eat and hunt, we never have to waste time thinking about these things again. Without habits, we'd have to recreate our behaviors every single day, from scratch. Like infants, we'd have to explore, test and sample every action, sensation and behavior before moving forward. We'd never get anywhere.

BRAIN TERRAIN

To really understand the challenge posed by learning, plasticity and habit, it helps to imagine the mountainous terrain of the earth. While the microscopic structure of the brain resembles a sculpted bush, its function resembles the weather-worn terrain of a rugged landscape. To get the idea, stand on a mountain top and notice how water has sculpted the terrain around you. Imagine the history and process of rut creation: a drop of water falls on a high place and starts making its way down, carving a very faint path as it goes. Later, another drop falls nearby and, seeking the lowest level, courses down the path set by its predecessor. After a thousand rainstorms, a channel is cut into the land. After a thousand years, a valley. After a thousand centuries, a canyon. Now the path of falling water is completely constrained. Any water that falls in the area will be channeled in the same direction.

The lessons here are severe and highly instructive. The first is obvious: the strongest habits and behaviors are those that are acquired early in life. Old ruts run deep, so whatever your skill, craft or discipline, you'll want get it right at the outset.

Second, if you want to re-route the flow and carve a new channel in your life, you're going to have to hike all the way back up to the crest of the mountain, to the origin of your habit, and start a new watercourse. This requires, like it or not, sustained intentional effort. The deeper the groove that you want to change, the more laborious the reps you're going to have to perform.

The dilemma now becomes clear: the human nervous system is both an incredible learning machine and a device that's prone to unconscious, habitual behavior. Grooves and ruts are essential for survival and performance, but they can severely limit what we can do.

This is the paradox of skill development: if you're not sufficiently grooved, your skills will be weak and wandering, but if you're too deeply grooved, you'll find it hard to do anything besides what you already know. The problem becomes obvious as soon as we try to improve our performance in some task, activity or sport. Skill development requires repetition, but repetition inevitably puts us at risk for getting stuck in habit.

PERSONAL METASKILL

The paradox of plasticity calls for a metaskill, a skill of revising habits, grooves and ruts. Arguably, this is the most important of all skills, and one that's particularly essential in our modern, alien environment. After all, anyone can carve a neural groove in childhood or young adulthood; we do this naturally, simply by repeated action. If we're lucky and diligent, we carve some functional grooves that we can depend on for the rest of our lives. But if the world changes or a groove takes us in the wrong direction, who among us can rewire our habits? And how do we do it?

RECOGNIZE AND REWIRE

The process, of course, begins with recognition. Habits are hard to see when you're deep in a canyon of highly conditioned behavior. This is why most teachers—athletic trainers, business coaches, consultants, counselors and therapists—advocate some kind of separation from the routine, mundane flow of daily life. In effect, they tell us to journey up to a high point where we can see the ruts, valleys and canyons of our personal and organizational experience.

Easy to say, hard to do. After all, who has the time to get outside the chronic emergency we call modern life? Most of us can scarcely manage the chaos as it is, much less journey to the mountain top for a better view. But the promise is real and the time will be well-spent. Even a glimpse of a deep and dysfunctional groove gives us an opportunity to change its course.

SLOW DOWN AND SENSE UP

Once we recognize a rut or groove, we're in position to transform the landscape of our habits. But the only way to really get out of a rut is to intentionally, slowly crawl back up to the ridge line of neural topography and start carving a new watercourse. Essentially, we need to take the time to go back to the beginning and start the groove all over again.

The best way to understand this process is to think about music education. You don't even need to be a musician to understand how it works: Week 1: Teacher assigns a song, a scale or a riff and the student goes home to practice. Week 2: Student returns and demonstrates his or her proficiency. Teacher says, "OK, that's pretty good. Let's try it again, only slower." And that's pretty much it, repeated over and over by thousands of music teachers around the world every day—a simple model for every other kind of skill training that we might want to engage in.

MONOTASK

Not only do we need to slow down, we also need to concentrate our attention directly on the desired groove, habit or rut in question. This means doing one thing at a time and only one thing. Unfortunately, the modern world also works against us. We are so often rewarded for doing many things simultaneously, monotasking strikes us an incredible waste of time. Nevertheless, it remains an essential requirement for habit revision. We absolutely must attend to the rut or groove that we're seeking to revise. Otherwise, we are really wasting time.

DO THE WRONG THING

Naturally, the challenge of habit reform gets more difficult as we grow older. We take comfort in familiar patterns and seek them out, deepening our habits further. In the process, we simultaneously become averse to new movements, new ideas, new challenges; we become increasingly neophobic.

To get out of our rut, we have to endure some unpleasant sensation and experience. Dan Millman, author of *The Way of the Peaceful Warrior*, described the challenge perfectly: "When you're doing it wrong, what's wrong feels right and what's right feels wrong." In other words, to get past the sticking point of habit, you're going to have to do the wrong-feeling thing for a time, maybe a very long time, until that wrong-feeling thing begins to feel right. If we're going to succeed in revising ruts and habits, we have to get comfortable with feeling uncomfortable.

DEEP, DELIBERATE AND MINDFUL PRACTICE

No matter what kind of habit you're attempting to develop or transform, concentrated effort is essential. Two recent books are particularly relevant for aspiring habit-crafters: Daniel Coyle's *The Talent Code* and Geoff Colvin's *Talent is Overrated*. Both writers are passionate advocates for concentrated engagement and skill development. Coyle tells us about the importance of "deep practice" while Colvin writes of "deliberate practice." No matter the label, the idea is the same: focused, dedicated, committed effort directed at performance training. This means full immersion and *work*. Not just reps, but high-quality reps. It's not enough to just drop in, dabble in the practice and head back to habit-land. No, we're looking for quantity, quality and mindfulness: attention to change and subtlety. Success demands complete commitment and mind-body participation.

CULTURAL METASKILL

As we've seen, individual habits wield immense influence over our behavior and ultimately, over the trajectory of our lives. But what happens when individual habit-forming brains link themselves together into vast cultural networks?

The same thing.

The mechanism may be different, but the principle is identical. That is, our cultural nervous system also exhibits "use-dependent plasticity." Ideas, memes and stories that are repeated tend to perpetuate themselves in deeper and deeper grooves. Patterns of thought, language, relationship and connectivity become entrenched and begin to span generations. Cultural forms become habitual.

As with individuals, cultural habits often play out unconsciously. The ideas, memes and stories that we supposedly "create" are often mere repetitions of forms that have gone before us. And when we repeat those ideas, memes and stories, we simply etch these neuro-cultural grooves deeper, making their perpetuation more likely. Naturally, this suggests that we look for a cultural metaskill, a process by which we can recognize and rewire the habitual patterns of thought and behavior that limit what we can do collectively.

Just as with individual habit, recognition is the essential first step to cultural transformation. This is where artists, journalists, historians, free-thinkers and outliers become so immensely valuable. These are people who have journeyed to a remote mountain top and surveyed the cultural landscape from an entirely different viewpoint. Standing above the terrain of cultural habit, they can see the ruts and grooves of relationship and ideas; they can tell us about our inclinations, our path and to some extent, our future.

Sadly, modern culture discourages the panoramic perspective and in turn, limits what we can know about ourselves. By placing ever more emphasis on specialists and specialized knowledge, we deepen our ruts and blind ourselves to the very understanding that might help us create change. Specialization is itself a rut, a groove that simply deepens itself.

Of course, recognition of cultural grooves is not enough. Just as with personal transformation, cultural habit reform is hard work that demands lots of repetition. Western civilization itself is a deep rut. Our habits of environmental domination, empire and destruction lie at the bottom of a deep cultural canyon. It's going to take a lot of uphill work to get to the ridge; as a culture, we're going to have to get comfortable with being uncomfortable.

Naturally, many of us will look to leaders, artists, visionaries, teachers, activists and trainers to step up and help us etch some new grooves in the cultural landscape. But as important as these high-profile leaders might be, anyone can play a role in rewiring cultural habits. Anyone can tell a new story, seek out a new meaning, promote a new orientation. Anyone can resist participation in dysfunctional cultural habits. Anyone can work uphill and start a new groove. All it takes is focused labor, mindful reps and deep deliberate practice.

GO TO THE MOUNTAIN

So go to the mountain. Take in the vista of your personal landscape and the cultural terrain that lies before you. Note the way the water flows. Note the rise and fall of the land, the shape of the watercourse and the direction of the flow. Study it and remember what you see.

Next time you're down in the valley of routine and habit, remember that view. If you're not flowing where you want to go, climb back up and carve a new groove.

EARTH LUST

If not for sex, much of what is flamboyant and beautiful in nature would not exist. Plants would not bloom. Birds would not sing. Deer would not sprout antlers. Hearts would not beat so fast. But ask an assortment of creatures, what is sex? and they will give you very different answers.

>Olivia Judson
>*Dr. Tatiana's Sex Advice To All Creation*

In the belly of the furnace of creativity is a sexual fire; the flames twine about each other in fear and delight. The same sort of coiling, at a cooler, slower pace, is what the life of this planet looks like. The enormous spirals of typhoons, the twists and turns of mountain ranges and gorges, the waves and the deep ocean currents - a dragonlike writhing.

>Gary Snyder
>*A Place in Space*

Don't worry, it only seems kinky the first time.

>Unknown

The first time I heard the Barefoot Sensei speak around a campfire, I was entranced. The Sensei is a powerful and authentic teacher, a visionary of body, land and foot. On this delightful summer evening in the Pacific Northwest, he delivered an intriguing set of stories, opinions and visions, most of them crafted around themes of bare feet, land, earth, training and activism. The conversation danced like the flames of the fire, light faded and stars appeared as the tribe gathered around. Stories came and went, but the Sensei held center stage.

After a string of compelling and often hilarious narrative, the Sensei became philosophical and began to speak of his personal dream and life path. He promised us that someday soon, he'd be "going back, deep into the wild."

We waited for more and passed the bottle around, anticipating the explanation that was sure to come.

"I'm headed out," he told us, "back into the wild. I've got everything I need. I'm going to foot the path into the wilderness and have an orgasm with the earth."

Suddenly, my attention jumped to a whole new level. Never having heard this expression before, my curiosity cried out. "Wait!" I nearly shouted. "What are you getting at? How can you have an orgasm with the earth? And more importantly, how can I have one?"

GETTING DOWN

Some will dismiss the Sensei's phrase as a bit of hippie hyperbole, a wildman fantasy with an erotic twist. But it's not. The Sensei has done it before and he fully intends to do it again. I have no doubt that this experience is real for him and for others as well. But still, we need to—excuse the language—go deeper and find out what this idea is all about. Undoubtedly, some of us may need an explanation and/or an instruction manual.

So the questions before us: What is an "orgasm with the earth?" What is this "earth lust?" Is it sex with the biosphere, our bioregion, this land, this habitat? Is it natural? Is it normal? How do we do it? And most importantly, is it hot?

What's that you say? You've never had an orgasm with the earth? You're kidding, right? Surely you must have at least done some heavy petting. You must have taken a backpack trip into the mountains or at least made a day hike to a high peak. You must have felt the summer breeze on your skin, the glow in your flesh and the intoxication of your spirit. If not, this is something that you must do, and soon.

If this all sounds preposterous, think again. When you get right down to it, sex with people and sex with the earth aren't really all that different. There's the romance, the anticipation, the first touch, the arousal and the immersion. There's the sensual contact and the virtuous circle of touching and being touched. There's a sense of safety, comfort, danger and exhilaration. The physical body comes forward, bringing deep primal memories and unification with all of life itself. If you can do one kind of sex, you can do the other.

MY FIRST TIME

For my part, I can vividly recall a number of earth-shattering earth-orgasms, mostly from my days as a climber in the mountains of California. Climbing, like many outdoor sports, is all about getting your body into intimate contact with the natural, tactile world. Exposure promotes vivid sensation, anticipation and engagement. Gravity provides focus and sharpens attention to the here and now. Tactile awareness deepens as fingers and toes probe for subtle variations in form and texture. Skin becomes alert and aware. Every sense comes alive, passionate, desiring ever more. Long summer days of perfect rock, perfect weather, powerful physicality and the sweet caress of a gentle breeze.

There was usually a climax of course, when we reached the safety and panorama of the summit, but this was but a single orgasmic moment surrounded by hours of caress and erotic pleasure. Even the moonlight descent, with our bodies dirty, bruised and fatigued by our efforts, was sensual magic, a feast for eyes, ears, skin and spirit. Only when we reached the highway would the spell be broken.

Later, I began to realize that climbing, for all its intensity, exposure and adrenaline, wasn't really necessary to achieve an earth orgasm. In fact, simply walking through the high country of Yosemite usually gave me a similar result. The intoxicating air of summer, the gently erotic curves of the granite domes, the sweet, fresh water that coursed down creek beds into soft inviting meadows, the subtle and revealing light that played across the alpine vistas: there was enough arousal here for anyone with sensation and attention. My skin, my senses and my spirit would always quicken in anticipation.

John Muir knew it all along of course, this sensual passion for the natural world, especially the Sierras:

> The grand show is eternal. It is always sunrise somewhere; the dew is never dried all at once; a shower is forever falling; vapor is ever rising. Eternal sunrise, eternal dawn and gloaming, on sea and continents and islands, each in its turn, as the round earth rolls.

FOR THE LOVE OF LIFE

For many, the popular archetype of Earth is female, and some might suppose that it's only men who would be lured into her arms. But when speaking of earth lust, there's no need to discriminate by gender, one way or the other. All people, of any sexual persuasion, can find erotic love in nature's embrace. Male or female, straight or gay, all can become passionate about the charms of the biosphere, land and habitat. Many call her "the goddess Gaia" and assume her to be female, but we can use any gender label we like. The biophilic impulse is really pan-sexual; we can all find pleasure here, no matter which pronoun we choose.

Of course, you might want to dismiss this entire line of inquiry as the lunatic raving of back-to-the-earth philosophers gone mad. But no less a figure than E.O. Wilson has championed a similar, slightly less erotic idea, one he calls *biophilia*. Wilson is no hippie or pornographer. In fact, he is a two-time winner of the Pulitzer Prize, a professor of Entomology at Harvard University and a fellow on the Committee for Skeptical Inquiry. Wilson is not a person given to rash, impulsive carnal speculation.

When all dressed up in asexual academic language, the term *biophilia* (literally "love of life") refers to our "innate tendency to affiliate with other living creatures and processes." Of course, Wilson wasn't explicitly erotic about his biophilia. (His views on sociobiology attracted enough controversy as it was.) But my guess is that if we could get him around the campfire in the company of a few friends and under the influence of the right libations, he would confess to knowing exactly what we're talking about.

When E.O. Wilson talks about biophilia, he's talking about a deeply physical, primal need for contact. Just as social animals have a strong need to maintain contact with one another, so too do we long to touch our living environment. What our bodies want is contact with plants, animals, rolling terrain and open sky. Our senses crave this stuff. We need to smell the land, touch the dirt with our bare feet, feel the textures of the plants, see the movement of the animals, and feel the wind on our faces.

Massage therapists often speak of the power of touch to promote human health. We know, for example, that infants who are touched frequently grow larger and healthier, while infants who are touch-deprived fail to develop normally. As social animals, we thrive on physical human contact, but there also seems to be an even wider need that goes beyond our species. We need to touch, smell and see living things of all varieties; in a sense, we need to massage and be massaged by the natural world. We need to be stroked by driving rain, blinding sun, steep terrain and long distances.

HEALTH AND BIOPHILIA

We now know that nature contact is a powerful driver of human health. Hospital studies show that patients with a window view of trees in a natural setting had shorter post-operative stays, fewer complications and requested less pain medication than those who had a view of a brick wall. And we have all heard about the beneficial effects of pets on sick human patients. It is obvious that contact with trees, dirt, rocks and animals is good for us.

In *The Biophilia Hypothesis*, Roger Ulrich cites studies analyzing the effects of outdoor scenes on stressed individuals. His findings suggest that "viewing unthreatening landscapes tends to produce faster and more complete restoration from stress than does viewing unblighted urban or built environments lacking nature." Apparently, natural settings tend to stimulate the parasympathetic nervous system, that branch of the nervous system associated with rejuvenation and tissue repair. One hospital study found that patients exposed to "serene" landscape pictures showed significant reductions in blood pressure. Another study suggested that patients responded more positively to wall art dominated by natural content, but tended to react negatively to abstract painting and prints. A prison study found that inmates with a view towards nearby farms and forests were less likely to report for sick call than those whose cell windows faced the prison yard.

PRIMATE'S PREDICAMENT

Sadly, one thing is obvious: we, as a people, are not getting enough earth sex and we aren't having enough orgasms with the biosphere. I have no way to quantify this claim, but I have no doubt that modern Americans are suffering an acute earth-sex drought. With millions of people chained to their desks, incarcerated in their cars and stressed to the absolute limit, it seems increasingly unlikely that people are having sex of *any* variety, much less passionate lust in the arms of the earth.

This may sound like an overstatement, but it actually constitutes a genuine public health emergency. After all, you probably know how it goes when you're going through a conventional sex drought: anxiety and frustration become acute, distraction becomes constant, health and exuberance begin to suffer. The urge to merge pushes itself into consciousness thousands of times each day. You can't work, you can't think and you're eventually forced into cheap alternatives that are completely without heart or soul. Similar symptoms are certain to arise when we go through an earthsex drought.

SEX ED

Unfortunately, our culture is suffering from an epidemic of erotic amnesia; we've forgotten our primal passion for the natural world. And even among those who have retained the simmering lust, the basic skills are often lacking. Obviously, it's time for some remedial education.

So let's begin at the beginning. First of all, you'll want to begin with the art of foreplay. The earth goddess doesn't reveal her charms without some seduction and effort. As Ovid wrote: "She will not come to you gliding through the yielding air; the fair one that suits must be sought…" You can't just show up and start fooling around; you'll need time for transition, anticipation, romance and seduction.

So set the time aside, away from the regular distractions in your life. Block off your calendar, protect some sacred space. Then, once you're committed, start your preparation. Pack the right clothes, assemble your provisions and plan your route. Set the mood and pay close attention to your lover. Be quiet and observant of detail.

As engagement begins, move towards embrace. If you're going to have an orgasm with the earth, you've got to put your body out there. You've got to expose yourself and make yourself vulnerable. You've got to be, in some sense, naked. This doesn't necessarily mean stripping off your clothing, although it might. What it really means is getting away from the thickest forms of urban insulation: the comfortable housing, the climate-controlled automobiles and all the electronic mechanisms that stand between our bodies and the body of the earth. Urban insulation, when carried to its logical conclusion, acts like a triple-layer condom, deadening sensation and making orgasm all but impossible.

Good earth sex is highly physical to be sure, but it's much more than mechanical intercourse. Sure, you can drop into nature in a helicopter or have a drive-by copulation on a cruise ship. You can fly over her gorgeous body in a small airplane or gawk at her wonders from the safety of a Land Rover. But while these methods may give you a quick burst of excitement, they lack commitment and intimacy.

In fact, most of our modern attempts to merge with the earth amount to little more than voyeurism or phone sex. Lacking time or interest in an authentic act of engagement, we simply cue up a nature special on the DVD player or dial in something on the Discovery Channel. And there we're treated to leaping whales, blood-thirsty predators, and the time-lapsed glory of Gaia's naked flesh, all with remote control in hand. After a few minutes, this action brings us to a pathetic faux orgasm and a return to the sports network or the refrigerator.

To have a truly meaningful orgasm with the earth, you've got to get your feet on the ground and your body into the outdoors. Intimacy means involvement. If you want to really get intimate, you're going to have to do more than click on a couple of hyperlinks. You have to be here, now. This means physical commitment and time.

Naturally, when it comes to earthsex, position is of supreme importance. The standard choices—deep valleys and high mountain ridges—are excellent of course, but don't limit yourself. Keep your mind open to terrain, light and landform. Anticipate the changing light, the flow of the clouds and weather, the changes in sound and the movements of animals. If a new position draws you, move towards it strongly, but without force. Keep listening and feeling your lover's moods; the land may suggest a new position, so be ready to adapt.

No matter the position, go towards your lover with a balanced physicality and spirit: strong-soft, powerful-adaptable, eager-patient. You are intent, you are passionate, you are absorbed. But you are also gentle, kind, compassionate and patient. You can be strong but you can yield, always deepening connection, contact and embrace of the divine. The more balanced your spirit, the more you can give, the more you can receive.

JUST DO IT!

As most people now realize, conventional sex is a powerfully health-positive experience. Even the most conservative medical publications tell us that sex relieves stress, boosts immunity, burns calories, improves cardiovascular health, boosts self-esteem and reduces pain.

The prescription is clear; sex is good for your health. It's even better if you do it with people you love. It'll lower your blood pressure, normalize your stress response, activate your parasympathetic nervous system and help you sleep. For these reasons, physicians now routinely advocate more sex for their patients.

Of course, most physicians are currently prescribing conventional sex with people and have yet to take things to the logical next level. But that may change. As more and more experts begin to understand the dramatically health-positive effects of biophilia and nature contact, they may very well expand their recommendations. They may just start telling their patients to spend more time in natural settings, getting their bodies into intimate contact with wild habitat, dirt, plants, animals, rocks and water.

It won't be long before they're writing prescriptions that say "Go outside and have an orgasm with the Earth."

"And call me in the morning."

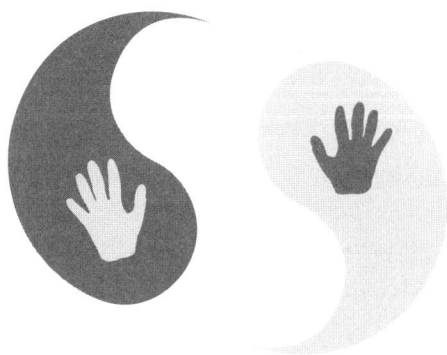

BAG OF TRICKS

Many native traditions held clowns and tricksters as essential to any contact with the sacred. People could not pray until they had laughed, because laughter opens and frees us from rigid preconception. Humans had to have tricksters within the most sacred ceremonies lest they forget the sacred comes through upset, reversal, surprise. The trickster in most native traditions is essential to creation, to birth.

> Byrd Gibbens
> *Far From Home: Families of the Westward Journey*

I not only want to describe the imagination figured in the trickster myth, I want to argue a paradox that the myth asserts: that the origins, liveliness, and durability of cultures require that there be space for figures whose function is to uncover and disrupt the very things that cultures are based on.

> Lewis Hyde
> *Trickster Makes This World: How Disruptive Imagination Creates Culture*

Without the laugh, there is no Tao.

> Lao-tzu

In 2006, former Vice President Al Gore gave us a compelling message in his landmark film, *An Inconvenient Truth,* the centerpiece in his campaign to educate citizens about global climate change. The documentary was a critical and box-office success, winning an Academy Award for best documentary feature. It has had a powerful impact all around the world.

The central message in *Inconvenient Truth* was troubling enough in its own right, but becomes even more so when we realize that climate change is only one planetary-scale inconvenience looming over our heads. The expanded list is both grim and familiar: population growth, habitat destruction, species extinctions, water shortages, topsoil erosion, destruction of fisheries and rainforests, social injustice and expanding militarization. All are threatening and all are growing with each passing day. And so, given the long list of afflictions that we now face, the documentary of our times really needs to be called *Inconvenient Truths*.

ACTIVISTS AND REVOLUTIONARIES

Gore laid down the challenge, but it is up to us to take it to the next level. His title suggests a strategy and an attitude: in a world of inconvenient truths, what we need more than anything else are *inconvenient people*. Inconvenient people are those who are willing to step up and challenge the dominant cultural paradigm that supports ill health, environmental destruction and social injustice. Inconvenient people are not content to receive their culture passively and without dissent. Inconvenient people ask hard questions and tell hard truths. They speak, create and act.

There are several varieties of inconvenient people in our midst. The first are polite activists. These people set up non-profits, sign a board of directors, raise money and start campaigns. Much of their work consists of signing up volunteers to do research, lobby, persuade and raise more money. These activists may be inconvenient thorns in the side of established powers, but they generally play by established rules. They work hard, but their progress tends to be incremental. Over time, many of these activists become "grinders," working long hours, fighting over detail, policy and procedure. Victories, when they come, are important, but rarely spectacular.

The activist's work is honorable, but is often ineffective. Power structures are stacked against change and non-profits are in a weak position to make things happen. Unfortunately, "dot org" is too often synonymous with "powerless and irrelevant."

When activists and non-profits run out of steam, some of us become frustrated and call for a more active form of activism. We come to the conclusion that what we really need are *revolutionaries*.

Revolutionaries are people who are willing to stand directly in the path of social injustice and environmental madness. They accept high levels of personal risk and challenge established hierarchies with direct language and in-your-face action. Revolutionaries are not patient people. In fact, they are *extremely inconvenient*.

Given the magnitude of our predicament, this style of action is both appropriate, meaningful and essential. Nevertheless, there is danger here: by the time passions get to this level, revolutionaries sometimes cross the tipping point into extremist ideology and in a paradoxical turn, ineffectiveness. Being a strident, passionate revolutionary is inspiring—when it works. But entrenched powers police their territories with great vigilance and are well-equipped to stamp out revolutionary ideas and revolutionaries themselves.

Revolution, especially in a paranoid, post-911 world, is an extremely high-risk proposition and the consequences of miscalculation can be dire. Revolutionaries run the risk of isolation and incarceration and in turn, the abrupt termination of their activism. This is not a path to be taken lightly.

There is another option here and that's to make a distinction between overt and covert rebellion. The overt revolutionary challenges power directly: he chains himself to the bulldozer or sets up camp in trees that are slated for logging. He sinks whaling ships and pulls up survey stakes. He talks loudly and carries a big monkeywrench.

The covert rebel, meanwhile, turns his efforts inward and makes a personal statement to the world at large. In this style, health itself becomes an act of rebellion. In a culture that drives people towards mindless destruction of nearly everything, physical vitality included, personal health stands out as a courageous act of defiance: "I am an animal and I will not submit to a media-driven culture of passive consumerism. I am an animal and I will not waste my health in the service of environmental and social destruction. I am an animal and I will not lie down while we destroy the last living shreds of the biosphere."

This approach adds an entirely new dimension to our study of healthy living. What is normally cast as a bland, harmless lifestyle practice now becomes a potently disruptive force. In this light, health has nothing to do with longevity, smooth skin and tight abs. Instead, it's about living in protest and derailing the pathologies of a earth-hostile culture. In this context, health is no longer neutral or safe. Rather, it's a statement of protest.

MEET THE TRICKSTER

Important as they are, activists and revolutionaries are not the only players in our game of personal and planetary transformation. There are other ways to craft effective, inconvenient and meaningful lives. One of the most promising lies with the path of the trickster.

The trickster has played a role in almost every culture; the archetype is a human universal. He or she appears in thousands of stories in various forms. He scandalizes, disgusts, amuses, disrupts, chastises, and humiliates yet he is also a creative force transforming the world, sometimes in bizarre and outrageous ways. In Native American culture, coyote plays the trickster and is well-known for his inventiveness, mischievousness, evasiveness and cunning. He's a practical joker, always playing with meaning, assumptions, prejudices, roles, hierarchies and power relationships.

In our modern world, many of us would describe the trickster as a "cultural creative," a person who refutes the standard narrative that culture is a static thing, carved into stone by the ancients. She rejects the assumption that culture is a thing to be received and replicated, never questioned or transformed.

Sadly, many of have been conditioned to simply receive and accept the culture that is handed to us. We spend our lives in dutiful replication of cultural memes, photocopying the rituals of former generations onto our offspring. The trickster on the other hand, sees culture as a canvas, a lump of clay, a process to play with. Think of the raw material! So many memes to work with! Ideas, stories, song, books, movies, theatre, language: all ripe for recombination, revision and regeneration.

Above all, the trickster is a questioner. She questions authority, expertise, power structures, culture and of course, herself. She questions categories and assumptions about what is possible. She questions the status quo and business as usual. She won't sit still when told that something is impossible or that transformation "just isn't realistic." Instead, she is always ready with the questions "Why?" and "Why not?"

Ultimately, the trickster is an athletic multi-disciplinarian who refuses to get bogged down into any one camp, box or pigeon hole. Her identity is fluid and her interests dynamic. Never one to get trapped in a single point of view or a single field of inquiry, the trickster always has one foot…somewhere else. Both a bridge-builder and a destroyer of bridges, her philosophy is dynamic and holistic. She pulls us out of our entrenched, boring, specializations and gives us a glimpse of an alternative world.

Tricksters do their work on several scales, from the audacious to the local and personal. You might see them hanging banners on large buildings or painting a "crack" on the face of the Glen Canyon Dam. You might hear about them dressing up as trees and animals at corporate shareholder meetings. You might read about them bidding up the action at government timber-sale auctions, buying up land to protect it. And you might see their *subvertising* in print and on billboards: corporate memes visually altered to reveal alternative meanings.

This is all honorable work, but small-scale trickery is vital too. A good trickster is an opportunist who looks for any chance to transform a dead meme or attitude into something more life-promoting. A conversational trickster can transform even a simple phrase and bring new meaning to mundane moments of life. These "tricks" may be invisible to almost everyone, but their power can be immense.

In philosophy and action, the trickster strikes a delicate balance of gravity and levity. She has no illusions about the severity of today's challenges, but refuses to be crushed under their weight. She understands the state of the biosphere and the threats to the future, but she also knows the danger of self-absorption and chronic seriousness. Yes, the situation is dire. Yes, the dangers are immense. And yes, the amount of suffering in this world staggers the imagination.

But none of this stands as reason for abandoning our exuberance or our vitality. On the contrary, it stands as reason for redoubling our enthusiasms, our humor and our levity. Our exuberance is the source of our creativity and in turn, our effectiveness. When faced with daunting and compelling challenges, we need *more* joyful living, not less. And so the trickster keeps a balance: the greater the gravity, the more she dances, laughs and plays. The more she feeds her body and spirit with joy, the more she can bring to the predicament at hand.

And so we begin to see the surprising power in trickery. Even if it "fails" in the grand scope of activism and planetary-scale transformation, it still succeeds in giving life to the trickster herself and those around her. If all trickery does is to maintain the outrageous health and exuberance of the trickster, then that may be enough. And, one never knows how far the ripples of trickery might extend; one good trick tends to inspire more of the same.

Ultimately, tricksters are visionaries and senseis. They have journeyed past the land of the ordinary and quested to the distant horizon. And because they see ahead, they are in position to direct and shape our attention. They bear witness to the dangers, challenges and rewards of our time. They draw attention away from the familiar, the conventional and the habitual. They show us alternatives. They point to human vitality. They point to the human bond with habitat, the land, the animals and the earth. They point to joy and love.

If you can see the way, become a trickster.

If you can't, seek out a wise trickster and look where she's pointing. That just might be your path.

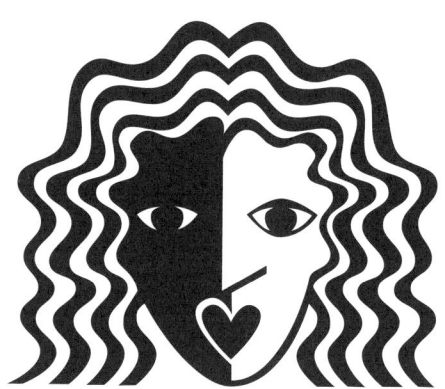

ACTION STEPS

The value of a book is not in the book, it is in the subsequent behavior of its readers.

Wendell Johnson

As our modern world grows increasingly complex, chaotic and interconnected, we often find ourselves wandering in confusion. A rising tide of information, alternatives and choices saps our energy, clouds our vision and distracts us from our ultimate purpose. To advance our health and activism, we need grounding and simplicity. As you go forward on your path, remember these general principles:

- Find a vigorous physical activity that turns you on and grow with it. The specifics are largely irrelevant. Simply find the movement art that you love, then follow this passion in an oscillating pattern of striving and rest. Make this process a priority in your life.

- Embed your body and spirit in the biosphere; learn the ways of your bioregion. Touch the world with skin, hands and bare feet. Expose your body to the forces of nature; make intimate sensory contact with the elements.

- Trust your nervous system: Your body is always looking for way to adapt and grow. You are resilient; you will rebound.

- Broaden your inquiry beyond your specializations: Look for connection and relationships between mind, body, spirit, land and tribe. Become a multi-disciplinarian.

- Bring your entire mind-body to your life, your work and your relationships. Thought and emotion are both essential to creative action.
- Define and refine your ultimate goals. Clarify your purpose and focus your power.
- Give and receive support: value and nurture your tribe. Exercise compassion and gratitude for yourself and those around you.
- Find a cause with meaning and fight for it.
- Find the play and humor in your body, your life and your relationships.
- When in doubt, dance.

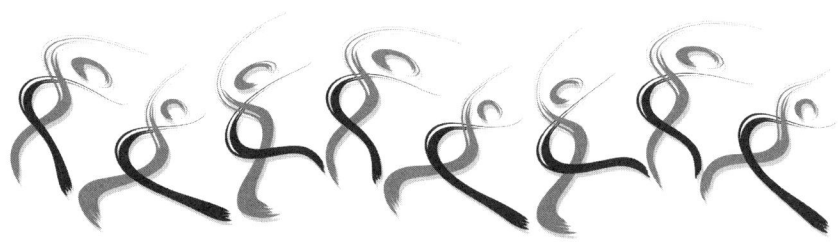

RECOMMENDED READING

Play: How It Shapes the Brain, Opens the Imagination, and Invigorates the Soul: Stuart Brown

Coming Home to the Pleistocene: Paul Shepard

Finite and Infinite Games: James P. Carse

Why Zebras Don't Get Ulcers: Robert Sapolsky

Opening Up: The Healing Power of Expressing Emotions: James Pennebaker

Rhythms of Life: The Biological Clocks that Control the Daily Lives of Every Living Thing: Russell Foster and Leon Kreitzman

Mirroring People: The New Science of How We Connect with Others: Marco Iacoboni

Muir: the collected nature writings of John Muir

Original Wisdom: Stories of an Ancient Way of Knowing: Robert Wolff

Learned Optimism: How to Change Your Mind and Your Life: Martin Seligman

Last Child in the Woods: Saving Our Children From Nature-Deficit Disorder: Richard Louv

A General Theory of Love: Thomas Lewis, Fari Amini and Richard Lannon

My Name is Chellis and I'm in Recovery from Western Civilization: Chellis Glendinning

The Language of the Land: Living Among a Stone-Age People in Africa: James Stephenson

The Age of Empathy: Nature's Lessons for a Kinder Society: Frans de Waal

Talent is Overrated: What Really Separates World-Class Performers from Everybody Else: Geoff Colvin

Wild: An Elemental Journey: Jay Griffiths

Descartes' Error: Emotion, Reason, and the Human Brain: Antonio Damasio

Sparks of Genius: Robert and Michele Root-Bernstein

Our Inner Ape: Frans de Wal

Omnivore's Dilemma: Michael Pollan

Emotional Intelligence and *Social Intelligence:* Daniel Goleman

The Comedy of Survival: Joseph Meeker

Pronoia: Rob Brezsny

Flow: Csikszentmihalyi

The Tao Te Ching: Lao Tzu

The Art of Happiness: The Dali Lama

Train Your Mind, Change Your Brain: Sharon Begley

The Old Way: Elizabeth Marshall Thomas

Sand County Almanac: Aldo Leopold

Exuberance: Kay Redfield Jamison

Tao Jeet Kune Do: Bruce Lee

Balance: In Search of the Lost Sense: Scott McCredie

Spark: The Revolutionary New Science of Exercise and the Brain: John Ratey

Waistland: The (R)evolutionary Science Behind Our Weight and Fitness Crisis: Deirdre Barrett

A Primate's Memoir: A Neuroscientist's Unconventional Life Among the Baboons: Robert Sapolsky

Narrative Medicine: The Use of History and Story in the Healing Process: Lewis Mehl-Madrona

Free Play: Improvisation in Life and Art: Stephen Nachmanovitch

Smart Moves: Why Learning is Not All in Your Head: Carla Hannaford

Mindset: The New Psychology of Success: Carol Dweck

American Idle: A Journey Through our Sedentary Culture: Mary Collins

Counter Clockwise: Mindful Health and the Power of Possibility: Ellen Langer

Deep Ecology: Living as if Nature Mattered: Bill Devall and George Sessions

Out of Our Minds: Learning to be Creative: Ken Robinson

Big History: The Big Bang, Life on Earth, and the Rise of Humanity: Big History: The Big Bang, Life on Earth, and the Rise of Humanity: David Christian (Teaching Company)

Biology an Human Behavior: The Neurological Origins of Individuality: Robert Sapolsky (The Teaching Company)

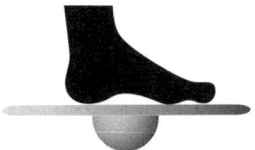

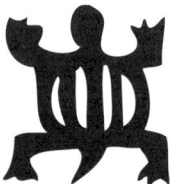

Change Your Body, Change the World

THE PRIMAL SCHOLAR

Frank Forencich graduated from Stanford University with a B.A. in human biology and neuroscience and has taught martial art, functional movement and health for over 30 years. He has traveled to Africa on four occasions to study human origins and the ancestral environment.

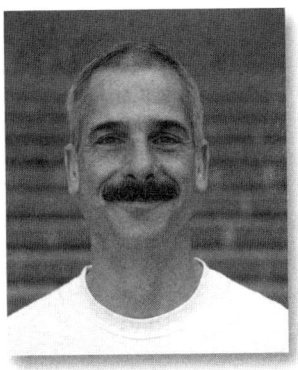

- Featured presenter: First Annual Conference on the State of Play Science, Stanford University, October 2008
- Guest lecturer: Stanford University Institute of Design, April 2009
- Featured presenter: National Applied Functional Physical Education Conference, October 2009
- Keynote presenter: American Alliance for Health, Physical Education, Recreation and Dance: Convention 2007
- Expert consultant to Wildfitness, UK
- Partner: National Institute for Play

Author of:

Play as if Your Life Depends on It: Functional Exercise and Living for Homo Sapiens

Exuberant Animal: The Power of Health, Play and Joyful Movement

The Exuberant Animal Play Book: Secret Moves and Games of the Play Masters

Contact frank@exuberantanimal.com

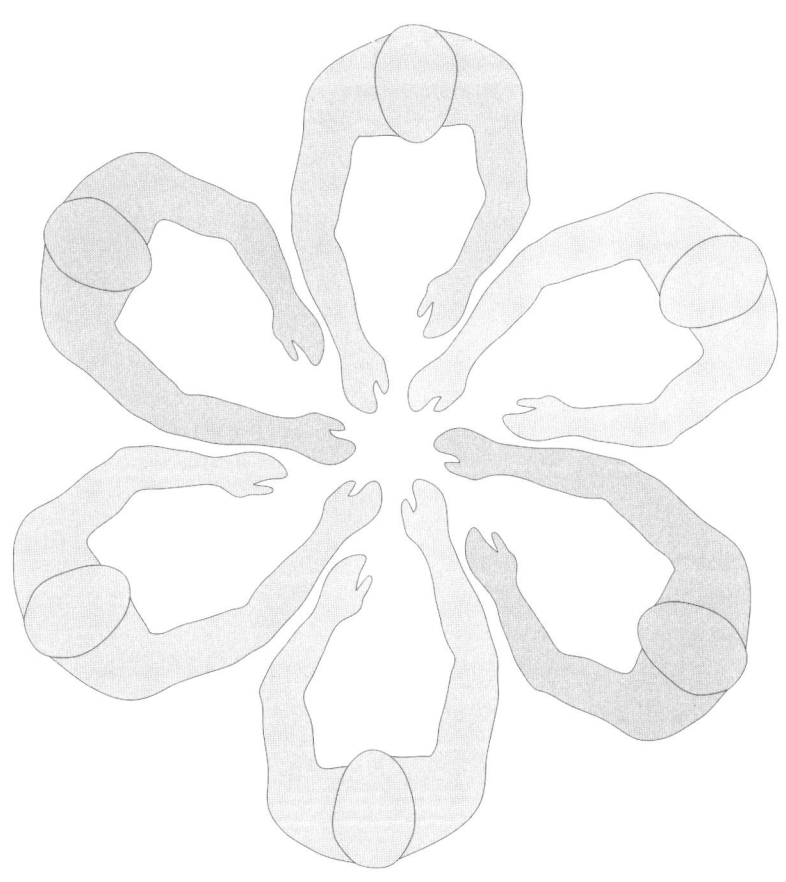

HEALTH, PERFORMANCE AND TEAM-BUILDING WORKSHOPS

Exuberant Animal® seminars are experiential training events dedicated to health education, performance, team cohesion and creativity. Each workshop is an integrated training experience that includes presentation and vigorous movement sessions. Participants discover new skills and ideas for improving their health, performance and social intelligence.

Ideal for managers, decision-makers, human resource directors, knowledge workers and health-care professionals.

- Increase team cohesion and good will
- Improve your understanding of good health practices and stress resistance
- Decrease health care costs, absenteeism and presenteeism
- Increase focus and concentration
- Increase creativity and innovation

You'll leave laughing, sweaty and inspired!

For complete information, see www.exuberantanimal.com

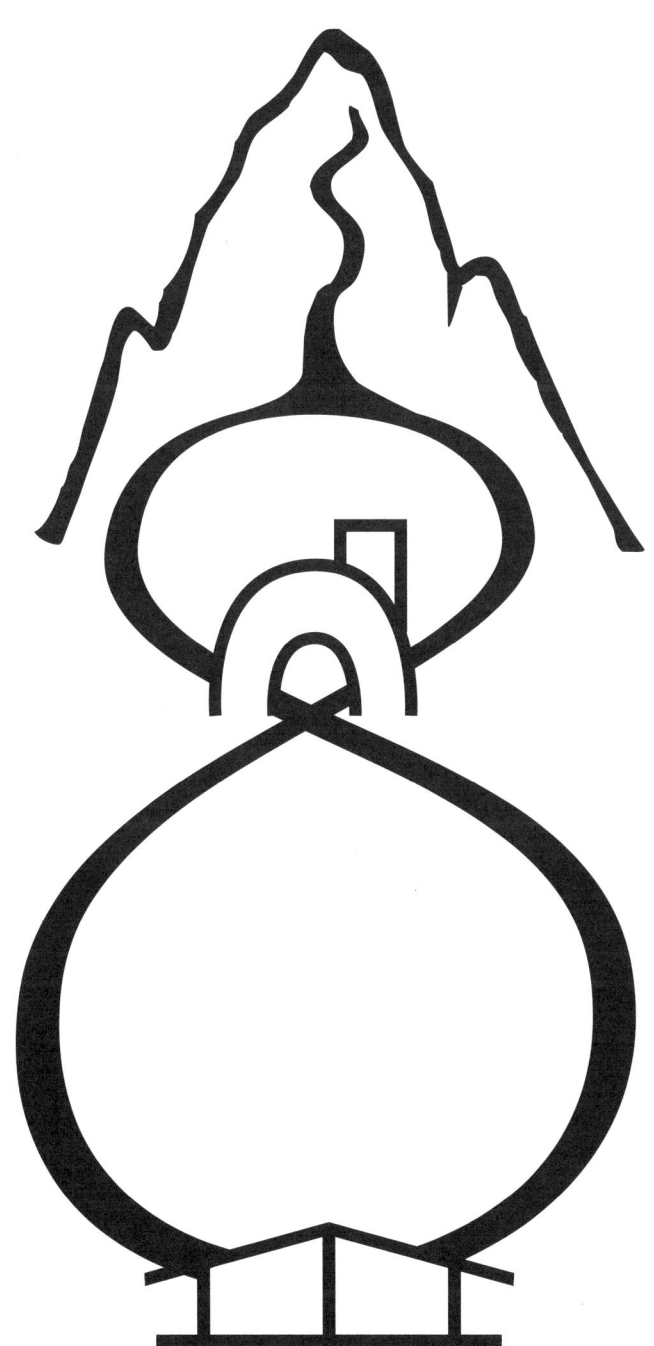

Change Your Body, Change the World